# A CASE OF THE F&$!#%K ITS!

## OVERCOMING MYSELF AFTER COVID-19 TRIED TO TAKE MY LIFE

# A CASE OF THE F&$!#%K ITS!

OVERCOMING MYSELF
AFTER COVID-19 TRIED
TO TAKE MY LIFE

KIA R. MERRIFIELD

Copyright © 2023 Kia Merrifield
All rights reserved.
To request permission, contact

Kia Renée Enterprises
1209 Hill Rd N #219
Pickerington, Ohio 43147
info@caseofthefits.com

Cover by Izabella Thomas
Paperback: 9798990821705
Ebook: 9798990821712
Printed in the United States
First Edition
Published by Kia Renée Enterprises
www.caseofthefits.com

*If you're silent about your pain,
they'll kill you and say you enjoyed it.*

**Zora Neale Hurston**

# TABLE OF CONTENTS

| | |
|---|---|
| **ACKNOWLEDGMENTS** | 8 |
| **FUCKING FOREWORD** | 9 |
| | |
| **SECTION I FUCKING HEALTH** | 10 |
| WHAT THE FUCK IS HAPPENING? COVID (2019 EDITION) | 11 |
| FUCK THE 2020 PANDEMIC | 13 |
| I FUCKING LOVE CAFFEINE | 15 |
| FUCKING EMERGENCY! | 17 |
| THREE FUCKING DAYS | 20 |
| YOUR FUCKING HEALTH IS MORE IMPORTANT! | 22 |
| | |
| **SECTION II THE FUCKING BACKSTORY** | 24 |
| WHERE DO I FUCKING BEGIN | 25 |
| WANTING FUCKING REVENGE | 29 |
| | |
| **SECTION III FUCKING MEN** | 34 |
| FUCKING JAMES | 35 |
| FUCKING FROGS | 40 |
| | |
| **SECTION IV FUCK JUDGEMENT** | 46 |
| FUCKING WEIGHT | 47 |
| FUCK THE BULLIES | 55 |
| FUCKING TRIGGERS | 59 |
| FUCK BEING SHY | 61 |

| | |
|---|---|
| **SECTION V FUCKING ADULTHOOD** | 64 |
| FUCKING COLLEGE | 65 |
| FUCK CANCER | 69 |
| FUCKING ROCK BOTTOM | 75 |
| FUCKING MOTHERHOOD | 77 |
| FUCKING FRIENDS | 84 |
| FUCKING ADVICE TO MY 25-YEAR-OLD SELF | 87 |
| WHO THE FUCK AM I? | 89 |
| GOING FUCKING FORWARD | 92 |
| **ABOUT THE AUTHOR** | 93 |
| **REFERENCES** | 95 |

# ACKNOWLEDGMENTS

I want to dedicate this book to God for sparing my life. I also want to pay tribute to my late father, T. Wayne Gatewood, who believed in me when I didn't believe in myself, and my late grandmother, Alberta Gatewood. Your strength and resilience are forever instilled inside me, and I miss you both dearly.

I am forever grateful to my husband, children, mother, and friends for their encouragement and tough love. I want to thank my sister Kerry, who can make me ugly cry by telling me to "get my ass up and get moving." My sister-in-law Amanda—thank you for your endless support and prayers, for becoming my unofficial editor, and for your responses to my endless emails and text messages telling me to "go deeper." My special cousins, Sharon and Rachel, thank you for being there for my children and me, and being my wise counsel when I am on the edge of the ledge. To my church family, no one supports me like my folks at Columbus Bible Way Church (CBWC). My friend Ed, you knew me when! Ha! You are the epitome of support, and I will never forget that. I love you all!

To the bullies and haters, old and new, I offer my thanks for providing the constant fuel I needed to keep going when I felt like giving up.

## FUCKING FOREWORD

I am feeling very nervous right now. People often think they know everything about those around them, like their family, friends, or the people they see daily. But the truth is: do we know everything about others? Do we know their background, where they came from, or what experiences shaped them? The answer is no. Even those closest to us may have hidden secrets, things they're ashamed of, or feel self-conscious about. When I started sharing my story, people often said, "I had no idea you struggled with that!" That's because I kept those parts of myself hidden, buried deep inside me, and never let anyone see them. But I decided to take off the mask, come out of the shadows, and be true to myself. It's a shame that it took me almost half of my life to do so, but I'm living my truth now. I feel anxious about sharing this, and I even joked with a friend that I'd need to be "pushed out of the plane without knowing" before I could share it with everyone. However, if it helps someone else, I'm willing to do it. Too often, we ignore, or avoid dealing with, our problems, especially in African American culture where it's often seen as a taboo topic.

# SECTION I
# FUCKING HEALTH

# WHAT THE FUCK IS HAPPENING? COVID (2019 EDITION)

Thanksgiving break in 2019 ended with the sudden onset of a fever on Sunday evening. I couldn't eat, was burning up, and was confused about what was happening. Monday morning, I dropped off my children and went to Urgent Care, where they told me they "thought" it was an upper respiratory infection because they had no other explanation after my strep and flu tests were negative. Then, I decided to work through it because my husband was working out of town, so I was the caretaker of our two small children. I relied on my family and friends to transport my children during this almost three weeks ordeal.

The fever came and went, and one morning I tried to get up but couldn't; it sounded as if I were underwater. I became nauseated and started sweating profusely. I called for my son, telling him to get his sister out of bed and ready for school. I tried navigating the bathroom and praying because I didn't know what else to do. I got the children to their destinations, drove to work, and sat in the parking lot, unable to muster enough strength to get out of the car. My very understanding and compassionate administrator saw my car and sent me a text telling me not to come into the building and to go and get some rest. Once I got home, I slept until 4 p.m., leaving just enough time to pick up my children.

The next day in my classroom—I am a Special Education Teacher—I was barely sitting up with my head propped up against the cabinet when my assistants, who are also my friends, made me go home. I honestly don't know how I cared for myself or my children during this time; my brave, then-six-year-old son had taken on the role of caregiver to his two-year-old sister, and he did a fantastic job.

It was the sickest I have ever been in my life, and I knew that this was much more than an upper respiratory infection. I was ill for almost a month, the worst of it being the cough that lingered on so badly, especially at night, that my chest felt like it was going to burst wide open.

**LITTLE DID I KNOW WHAT THE FUCK WAS TO COME.**

## FUCK THE 2020 PANDEMIC

In January 2020, we began to hear things about this virus: Coronavirus or Covid-19. All they said was that it was highly contagious, and it caused panic worldwide. I remember China being the new focal point, and I paid too much attention to it. In March, they began closing schools and businesses, causing people to lose their jobs due to layoffs. Everybody was in a panic. On March 13th, our governor announced that schools would be closed for a few weeks, which became almost a year. On July 18th, my husband said he wasn't feeling well and had a sinus headache that lingered for days. We decided to call the PCP, and he took us to the Covid test center to test my husband. We were all tested, and we both tested positive.

My symptoms were headache, shortness of breath, and a cough. I did not have a fever, but I was exhausted. My husband had a fever of 102 to 103°F depending on the day. He began hallucinating; he was unaware of his surroundings, which scared me. I called the emergency squad and when the paramedics arrived they checked all his vitals. My husband was so confused, and he kept asking me where he was going—I told him, "To the hospital." He did not know why I explained that he had a fever and was sick.

Once the paramedic took his vital signs, he told me that unless my husband was short of breath, honestly and indeed, he was better off at home because if he went to the hospital he would only sit there. After all, they were only taking the sickest patients. So that's what I did. I kept him home and cared best for him, and our two children, myself.My husband has underlying health issues, and I kept asking him if he was OK and if he could breathe. I was very thankful that the shortness of breath was not one of his symptoms, but he was as sick as I was in November 2019.

One thing that stands out to me was one morning, while we were sitting on the edge of the bed, he said, and I quote, "I talked to your dad last night." That scared me so badly because my father passed away on May 29, 2015. My heart dropped because I thought that moment he was going to die. I had heard the Governor of New York talk about seeing his dead relatives and having conversations with them while he was sick. My husband began to tell me what he and my father talked about, and he then looked at me, pointed to the hallway, and said, "You don't see him standing there? He's got on a brown suit and brown shoes," and this was just so crazy to me because my father had owned a brown suit and brown shoes.

All I could do was pray for my husband to be OK because I thought it was the end for him. He went through hell for fourteen days and then another fourteen days of the lingering effects, i.e., the cough that never goes away, and makes you feel like you've been a smoker your entire life. The pandemic sucked big time. We were all inconvenienced in the worst ways. Our children were remote learning, meaning they were home, people lost loved ones, etc.

In Ohio, schools did not resume in-person learning until April 2021, after being closed since March 2020 due to the Covid-19 pandemic. The concept of remote work was not widely accepted by employers prior to the pandemic, but it has since become the norm in many industries. My family faced significant challenges during this time due to both my health issues and my husband's job situation. After being laid off from his out-of-state job, my husband unexpectedly returned home and stayed with us for eighteen months. Despite the difficulties we encountered, we felt grateful that we were able to manage our finances and keep our household running with the help of God's grace. This unexpected turn of events allowed my husband to rest and recover, while also giving us a precious opportunity to bond as a family and grow closer together.

## FUCK COVID!

## I FUCKING LOVE CAFFEINE

I am a bona fide tea drinker. I have never liked coffee, and during my school years I loved to drink Tazo Awake tea, a black tea that tastes malted and is incredible.

When the pandemic hit, I began drinking two teas per day. I would purchase the 48-count box of tea bags, so I didn't have to continue running back and forth to the store. So, I did not think anything of it, but at the beginning of November I started to feel very jittery, as if I was having a panic attack, and I could not understand why. I began to get a headache; my ears hurt so bad that I thought I had an ear infection, and then I felt the worst. I got a cough again, so I was Covid tested and then I did a Telehealth visit, during which I was diagnosed with a sinus infection and got treated for it.

A few weeks passed, my ears weren't hurting, my headache was going away, and I didn't feel like I had a post-nasal drip; the doctor stated that I was having shortness of breath, probably due to some mucus drainage getting into my lungs. She gave me albuterol. The only time I've ever been short of breath is when I've been sick, which was years ago, with an upper respiratory infection and at one point bronchitis. I've never had asthma. I've never had any issues with breathing, so to have shortness of breath after the sinus infection went away, I couldn't understand what was going on.

Fast forward to December 4, 2020; I felt very anxious all day. I told my sister my anxiety level was through the roof, and I did not know why I thought that I couldn't calm myself down. My heart was racing, so I decided to make a trip to Urgent Care. I arrived at Mount Carmel Urgent Care at about 8:20 p.m. I was the last patient; the doctor asked what was happening.

I told him that I was having dizziness, shortness of breath, and ringing in my ears, and he did an EKG (an electrocardiogram). The doctor said, "Our machine is kind of wonky, but everything looks fine; just lay off the caffeine." The nurse printed out my information and sent me on my way. For the next few days I was still short of breath, but I laid off the caffeine.

At work on Wednesday, teaching virtually from home, I took a puff of my albuterol and a sinus pill because I was starting to have some drainage. I felt as though my heart was pounding out of my chest. I thought I couldn't catch my breath and, even after sleeping for the night, my heart rate was over 120 beats per minute.

I dropped my daughter off at childcare on Thursday morning but still felt horrible. At home I was so winded that I walked up the stairs and grabbed the first thing I saw to hold onto. I heard static, as if listening to the radio on the wrong station. I found out later this meant my brain was starting to lose oxygen.

I was sweating profusely; I could not catch my breath. My husband entered the hallway, and I told him I was going to the ER because something wasn't right. I decided to try to get through my morning Zoom session, but when I got on with my students my assistant looked at me and said, "You need to go now." So, I made the arrangements, got in the car, and went to the emergency room. I drove myself to the closest emergency room, ten minutes away. I would later learn that driving myself to the hospital could've ended in tragedy.

**GET FUCKING HELP IMMEDIATELY IF YOU DON'T FEEL WELL!**

## FUCKING EMERGENCY!

I got out of the car, and I could barely make it to the door. I stopped at least five times before I reached the desk and told the gentleman what I needed. He told me to have a seat. The nurse came and got me and took me directly to the back—once there, they did the EKG. They initially thought I had a heart attack, but after a chest X-ray, they were wrong. Nothing could've prepared me for what the doctor would tell me. "You have blood clots in your lungs, and we must admit you to the hospital." The look on my face overshadowed the tears dripping down my cheeks. I couldn't believe what I heard and needed a moment to gather my composure.

The doctor told me she would give me a moment because I needed to call my husband. We were in an actual life-or-death situation. I called my husband, with tears, and told him I was being admitted to the hospital for a pulmonary embolism, or blood clots in my lungs.

I sent my mother, sister-in-law, and sister a message to inform them of what had just happened. I began to pray that I was going to be OK.

Everything that went through my mind involved my children and my husband. I was forty-four years old, and I had just been diagnosed with blood clots in my lungs and signs that I'd also had a heart attack, when, in fact, my heart became enlarged due to the number of clots that filled my lungs.

Once I regained my composure, the Black emergency room doctor, Dr. Joyner, came in and told me that she was "thankful" that I listened to my body because most people don't, which ends tragically. I asked to be transferred to Riverside Hospital because I knew that they were, and still are, the best when it comes to heart issues, but I was so confused as to how I would be having heart issues when I had no signs.

God intervened once again. The Riverside emergency department was not responding. Dr. Joyner asked where I wanted to go, and I had to answer quickly. I told her, if I had to, I would go to Ohio State. Still, Riverside was my first choice.

A few moments later she retired and said, "It's time to go." I thanked her through tears, and she told me to improve. I had a reasonably pleasant experience on my ride to the hospital: the medic who rode in the back with me was a very nice, polite woman, and we talked about blood clots and Covid-19 and all the issues. I thanked her and the driver for their frontline service.

Once at the hospital, everything went so fast. I remember being very hungry, and tired because I was struggling to breathe so much that I was placed on oxygen. Once in my room, I was whisked away for a battery of tests: echocardiogram, CAT scan, drawing so many tubes of blood that I lost count, and a temperature check-up.

When I finally found a place to settle, I immediately called my husband via FaceTime. As soon as the video call connected, I could see my children's faces on the screen, and it was the first time I had seen them since I left earlier that day. I still remember the look on my son's face as he peered into the screen, and it broke my heart. He asked me when I was coming home—I told him I didn't know. Tears welled up in his eyes, and I knew he was scared. I tried to comfort him as best as I could, and told him that it was OK to cry. My daughter, who was still very young, didn't quite understand what was happening, but she wanted to know where Mommy was because they both thought I was at CVS Pharmacy. All I could tell them was that I was OK and that I would be home soon.

My husband was also on the call, but he was keeping his emotions in check. I could tell that he was scared, even though he would never say it aloud. We both knew that the future was uncertain, and we would need all the strength we could muster to get through this difficult time. We leaned on our faith, knowing that it would guide us through the storm and illuminate the path forward as we navigated the uncertain road ahead.

**FUCK!!**

## THREE FUCKING DAYS

And for the three days I was in the hospital, I was poked and prodded. The first day, I was unable to move because the cardiologist did not want the blood clots to travel to my heart. I sat in bed with my iPad and sent assignments and memos to my students. I was still trying to do my job. I said, "Well, I'm in the hospital, but I have what I need, so I can go ahead and continue to teach." It wasn't until I read an article about a teacher whose house was on fire that I decided against it. He continued to teach his students by using his neighbor's Wi-Fi outside while his house was in flames.

After reading that and speaking to my assistant, I decided it was not worth it. My family depended on me, and if something happened I was replaceable, so I left my work alone and decided to spend a little time with Jesus because I was so scared that I didn't know what else to do.

So, the second day, they decided to do a procedure called a thrombectomy, in which they took a catheter through my groin and were able to suck out the clots in my lungs. I wanted to see it, the surgeon showed it to me, and I lost count at twenty clots. I asked if they had got them all, and he told me that there was no possible way to cut the branches of my lungs, so they would put me on blood thinners to dissolve the remaining clots. That way, my heart would be able to begin to heal and pump correctly.

I could not believe what was going on. It was just strange to me, and it was like something out of a movie because I have only been in the hospital three times, to have my children and to have surgery. While in the hospital, I talked to my cardiologist, who said they were starting to see people develop blood clots due to the coronavirus. I still, almost four years later, have long-term Covid-19 effects on my memory; the brain fog is real. I remember telling him, and my sister, that my cycle changed, and I thought I was going through menopause. Now, there are studies showing that women's menstrual cycles were altered as a result of having coronavirus, so there is no telling what the long-term effects will be on all of us as a result of this virus.

**FUCK COVID AND FUCK THAT JOB!**

# YOUR FUCKING HEALTH IS MORE IMPORTANT!

The dismissal of the Urgent Care doctor at Mount Carmel could have cost me my life. Why are Black women not taken seriously when we are in pain or distress?

The dismissal of Black women by doctors is a well-documented problem in healthcare worldwide, stemming from systemic racism, and biases within medical institutions. This issue often leads to Black women receiving inadequate care, incorrect diagnoses, delayed treatments, and worse health outcomes compared to white women. It underscores the pressing need to tackle systemic racism and biases in medical institutions, as Black women frequently face barriers in accessing timely and appropriate care, resulting in serious consequences for their health. Implicit biases among healthcare providers significantly contribute to the dismissal of Black women's health concerns. These biases, influenced by societal stereotypes, can lead to dismissive attitudes and insufficient care. Stereotypes like the "strong Black woman" notion may cause doctors to overlook or downplay Black women's pain and symptoms, resulting in delays in diagnosis and treatment.

Additionally, historical instances of medical exploitation and mistreatment have fostered deep distrust of the medical establishment among Black communities. This distrust can discourage Black women from seeking care and worsen healthcare disparities. Communication barriers and cultural differences between Black patients and predominantly white healthcare providers worsen the problem. Black women may feel unheard or misunderstood by their doctors, leading to frustration and disengagement from the healthcare system.

Moreover, structural factors such as socioeconomic disparities and residential segregation disproportionately affect Black communities, contributing to poorer health outcomes. These systemic inequalities intersect with gender-based discrimination, further marginalizing Black women in healthcare settings. Addressing these challenges requires comprehensive efforts to dismantle systemic racism and biases within healthcare systems. Healthcare providers need cultural competency training to recognize and address implicit biases. Additionally, initiatives to enhance diversity among healthcare professionals and promote patient-centered care are crucial to ensure equitable and inclusive healthcare for all, regardless of race, or ethnicity.

**FUCK BIASED HEALTHCARE!**

# SECTION II
# THE FUCKING BACKSTORY

## WHERE DO I FUCKING BEGIN

I remember in elementary school, about second or third grade, I told one of the counselors that my uncle had touched me. I never heard anything else about it. I just remember feeling like, *damn, I've told them what he is doing to me,* and nothing was done, so I went on not saying another word about it, until one day my little brother and I were playing and I mentioned to him that Uncle D.S.M. was touching me. My brother is three years younger than me so he was about four or five at the time. He didn't understand what was being said. At a family cookout, weeks later, I know he approached my uncle and said, "Leave my sister alone." My uncle said nothing and walked away.

I belonged to a youth group at my church, and one evening we had some women come and speak about abuse and other issues that teenagers faced. One of the women said if anyone wanted to discuss anything in private that we could. After waiting to see if anyone else would get up, I went to the bathroom and entered one of the classrooms. I talked to the woman and told her what was going on with my uncle, and nothing ever happened: my parents were never notified.

I went into high school and didn't say anything to teachers or counselors. I had learned through health class and sexual education, and Planned Parenthood that what my uncle had done to me wasn't molestation—it was rape! Around my sophomore year in high school I befriended a girl I knew from middle school. We became best friends, and I confided in her later that year.

When I graduated from high school, I met a man named James and we became great friends. Eventually, I fell in love with him. During one of our conversations, he told me that I was hurting inside and needed to talk about it. I didn't want to talk about it, especially with a man. I was very reluctant, and it took months of him begging and pleading, but I told him what happened to me as a child.

I had moved from my parent's house into my first apartment during this time. Day in and day out, I would lie across my bed talking to him. I told him how one night, while my uncle babysat for my siblings, he made me watch him and his girlfriend have sex, and once she left, he made me do those same things to him. I told him about how, when we spent the night at my grandmother's house, he would have me in the bed with him under the covers and have intercourse with me while my female cousins were on the floor watching television in the dark. This went on for about four years, off and on, and I told him how alone I felt and that I wasn't protected.

I was angry because I felt that my parents should have known, and being violated at such a young age made me feel like damaged goods to men. After hours of me spilling my deepest, darkest secrets, he confided in me as well, about his own molestation. His firsthand knowledge of the situation made him very compassionate and supportive towards me, making me love him even more.

A few weeks later, James told me I needed to talk to my parents about what had happened. I was scared, which I shouldn't have been: I was an adult, but I was, nevertheless. So, one afternoon, I did it. I called my parents' home, and my mother answered. I told her I was thinking of taking the family on the Jerry Springer or Maury Povich show because I had a secret to tell. She told me to tell her, so I blurted it out, "D.S.M. raped me." My mother hung up the phone. In shock, I called back, and my cousin answered the phone and told me that he had molested her as well. I heard my mother in the background, and my cousin asked her why she hung up on me: she said I was lying. I was devastated. I couldn't believe that my mother, of all people, would say I was lying about such a horrific act.

James called later that night, and I cried and cried to him about whether my own mother would not believe me. He listened and told me he would be there for me through the ordeal. My father called me that night, asking me why I never said anything. He also wondered why he hadn't seen my uncle at family functions. From that point on, I had a very different relationship with my parents, especially my mother, because she did not believe me throughout the years. My father and I would have conversations, and one day I asked him why he never went after my uncle or did anything after I told him that I'd been raped. He told me, "You have no idea how it feels to think you protected your children, then to find out you didn't." I would not understand this statement until I became a mother. My parents did their best with the tools they had at the time.

I will not begin to tell their stories because they are not mine to tell, but I will say this: when you have multiple children—when I say multiple, I mean more than you can handle (for me it was two, for other people it could be ten)—especially if you're raising them by yourself, people get lost in the sauce and left behind, and things happen. Family secrets and generational curses take place that the mother and/or father may, or may not, be aware of.

It took me until I had children to really forgive my mother for her disbelief. I was very self-righteous with how I addressed her because I felt she should've known. It was her duty as my mother to know that something was wrong with me; I used to cut my hair in elementary school. I was angry, and I remember telling a counselor at school, not the entire story but I gave her some background. I'm not sure if there was a mandated reporter law back in the 80s, but I gave her some information, and nothing was done with it. I didn't disclose it to any of my friends until high school, but this was the first person I had told as we had a semi-relationship. I was not prepared for what was to come.

**FUCK BEING SILENT, TELL YOUR TRUTH!**

## WANTING FUCKING REVENGE

It was now out in the open, and I thought that meant my uncle would have been killed by nightfall. Not at all, he is still living and breathing to this day. A couple of years passed and I lived back home with my parents. I told them I wanted to press charges for rape—my mother told me that if I did, I would no longer be a part of the family. Once again, I was devastated and in disbelief over the fact that she wanted to protect the "family" instead of seeing justice served for her daughter. I told my parents that I felt I would never have a "normal" relationship with a man because of what happened.

After feeling defeated, I left things alone until 2005. I had so much anger and rage inside of me, and I decided that he had to pay for taking my innocence. I talked to a friend about this rage, and she suggested that I confront those I was angry with to begin healing. I decided to write a letter to my rapist D.S.M. In the letter, I told him of how he violated me and the trust of his sister and brother-in-law. How I would press charges against him if he didn't respond to my letter within five days. Well, five days passed and there was no response. I sent another letter. This time the letter was addressed to his wife: I told her that the man whom she had married was a child rapist, and that she needed to be aware for her grandchildren's sake—the girls and boys, because I heard that he had become partial to little boys as well. A month later, I still had no response, so I left it alone . . . again.

By this time, I had left home and gone to college. I decided to visit my parents for the weekend and decided that it was time for my father and I to sit and have a conversation about things, and I asked him the hardest question I had ever asked. Why didn't he protect me? Why didn't he kill him once he found out? My father was taken aback: I could tell by his expression. He told me that he didn't know what happened and that we wouldn't have been over at my grandmother's house if he had known. He also told me that he felt he did a decent job of protecting his children, and that I had no idea how it felt to know he had failed to protect me. Hurt filled his entire face. I felt bad because he was upset about it.

I asked my mother the same questions: she didn't know, and if my father had done something to him and gone to prison, how would she have raised us? My response was, "Women raise children alone every day."

My father told me that God had gotten him for everything he had done, but still, that wasn't good enough for me—I wanted blood.

One Sunday afternoon, my sister called to tell me my uncle was at my grandmother's house, so I hopped into the car and raced across town. Just as I turned the corner onto her street, he and his wife were driving off: he looked me right in my face, looked away, and kept driving. I followed them until they were a few blocks away from their house. I then called my sister, who told me I needed to let it be.

I turned around and headed back to my parents' house, found the phone number of the police department, and called to find out what, if any, recourse I had against my uncle.

The officer politely told me the statute of limitation was up. I was now twenty-eight and would have had to file charges no later than when I was twenty-one. I hung up the phone and burst into tears. How could this have happened? He was scot-free. I began having dreams about hurting him physically, confronting him. I was told that I could end up in jail if I did something to him. It would be months later, and in very different circumstances, when I would see him again.

In December 2005, my favorite uncle, Eliot, passed away. I saw D.S.M. at the funeral, which was expected: he was his brother. I had every opportunity to confront him, but I'd be behind bars if I had. Instead, I returned to my apartment in Fairborn, saying nothing.

Let's fast forward to July 2019. My maternal grandmother passed away, and we were at our church for her repass. I had a horrible heaviness in my chest and so much anxiety I felt like I could not breathe. It wasn't because my grandmother had passed away, because, if I am being sincere, I had an indifferent relationship with her as well, but she is no longer here, so we will not dwell on that. I came out of the church and saw my uncle standing next to my car, and in my mind, I thought, *this is now or never*, so I got on the phone and called my husband, and told him what I was getting ready to do. He said, "Are you sure?" I said, "Yes!"

I asked D.S.M. if he could step into the car. Could I talk to him for a moment. I was shaking so badly, nervous and anxious, and sick to my stomach, but this was it—I had to do it. It was the time. If I didn't do it now, it wasn't going to happen. He got into the car and willingly locked the doors, and I immediately told him that he looked like shit, and he looked like he had been through hell. He said he had been. I told him I remembered everything he did to me and made me do.

He said he did not recall, but was sorry if he did something like that. He also referred to his daughter, stating he did something to her but did not remember that either. It seems like a pattern: you harm someone and then conveniently forget about it. I went on to tell him how he tried his best to break me, of the hell I have been through in my life, and although he tried, he couldn't break me.

I told him I had a loving husband and children that he would never meet and that I prayed that God has mercy on his soul. He got out of the car, and that weight that I felt went from me. I remember driving to my mother's house afterward, screaming in my car like a banshee. I felt so much better, and I knew it was something that I could not have done when my grandmother was living. I told my family what I had done. One of my cousins thought it was inappropriate that I did it at that time, but I did not care because it was not for anyone else. It was for me. I called my husband and told him everything went well. He asked me how I felt now. I told him I felt lighter, and that is when I started to break free of that shame and filthiness.

So many times, especially in Black households and families, things are swept under the rug, resulting in generations of people being abused, brutalized, and not able to understand why certain things happen. I made it my business, before I even had children, that I was going to be the one to break the cycle, this vicious cycle, because after finding out about my other two cousins, I found out that more family members had been touched or raped by other uncles and cousins.

I prayed before I even got pregnant that my children would never experience this. I prayed that they would be protected and able to discern if they felt uncomfortable about someone, anyone, whether they were family or not. I prayed that if someone tried, they would scream bloody murder and fight, right then, so that they would not carry the weight of the shame, embarrassment, and guilt for years.

I explained this to my husband before we got married, and it was difficult for him to understand, but that was OK because I was going to make sure, as their mother, that this would not happen if I could help it. My son was about three and said one of his friends asked him to keep a secret. I overreacted and told him there are no secrets, and if anybody asked you to keep a secret, tell them secrets are bad. Now, he did not understand why I was saying that, and even now that he's eleven, he'll say things about secrets. Although I'm not as abrasive as I was when he was three, I still tell him and my daughter that if anyone wants them to keep a secret they should let me and their dad know, because secrets are not good.

In January 2017, I found out that I was pregnant with a girl. Although I was happy, I was also afraid of having a daughter. My husband could not understand why I felt that way, so I explained my reasons to him. I still pray every day to keep my child safe no matter what, and I tend to be overprotective, especially when it comes to my daughter. As a mother, I am like a protective mama bear with both of my children, but with my daughter I am even more vigilant.

One of my friends brought it to my attention that being too aware can sometimes bring the very things into existence. So, I had to change my thinking and just thank God for protecting my children completely, over and repeatedly. I even had a conversation with a friend who also has a daughter. She's very protective and wants to make sure it doesn't happen to her daughter, but every time she goes somewhere, she says to "make sure nobody touches your vulva." The daughter got mad. I know that was an opportunity for me to tell her, "You said it, she understands it, and leave it at that because you're beating a dead horse, and it can cause it to backfire."

No one wants to talk about the aftereffects, the remnants of sexual abuse or violation—people go one way or the other. You are either completely closed off sexually, or you are promiscuous. You feel you need to find love by any means necessary. Some people become people pleasers, and some people become sexual predators themselves. Depression, anxiety, self-harm, and addiction to things are aftereffects of being sexually violated. Of course, in 2024, more people have spoken out, and I'm so glad, but so many people still carry these secrets. Some people have gone, or will go, to their graves with the secret.

Get the therapy, confront them if you can, get yourself healthy now!

**FUCK BEING A VICTIM, I TOOK MY POWER BACK!**

## SECTION III
# FUCKING MEN

## FUCKING JAMES

Twenty-five years before *Love After Lockup* there was James and Kia. Disclaimer: James is not his real name.

I went through a period of meeting men, and sleeping with them was not always safe. I remember keeping a running list of partners with their names, birthdays, and other identifying information. Each year, this list became longer and longer without thinking.

My first experience with reciprocated love was with James, an incarcerated man. I learned so much over the thirteen years I was with him. I learned that a relationship is defined in one form, and we have friendship, mutual respect, love, and more love. I kept our relationship a secret for years because I didn't want to hear the negative comments. It was open season when I decided to be open about it with friends and family. Everyone thought I was crazy. I didn't care; I loved him. I would have moved mountains to be with him: the feeling was mutual. I felt as if he was my guardian angel, so to speak; he gave me a voice regarding my rape that no one else had given me, and he motivated me to strive to be better.

I couldn't wait to tell him when something good happened or what I had accomplished that week. He loved me when I didn't love myself and put up with my ever-changing moods and attitudes. My life with him was something that only those who experienced the same type of love understand.

This story is crazy, but if you want to hear it, here it goes. I graduated from high school in 1995, and during that time they used to publish all the Black graduates in the *Call and Post*. It was awesome because I saw myself in the newspaper; you thought you were famous. I had no idea that the *Call and Post* would change my relationships and how I viewed men.

One day I got a letter out of the blue from somebody I didn't know. I read it and tossed it aside, thinking nothing about it. I showed it to my mom. She's like, "Oh, he's in prison." Like what? I didn't know anybody in prison except my uncle (but not that uncle!), so I threw the letter away. Boy, oh boy, curiosity killed the cat. I got the letter out and decided to respond about a month later.

He had written to me looking for a pen pal and, since I had nothing better to do, I began writing to him regularly while continuing with my daily life. I decided that there was nothing wrong with it—we were friends. Whatever, about a year into it, we started to get closer. At this point, I didn't know anything. I was nineteen years old and started talking to him over the phone. Boy, phone bills increased quickly, but I was having fun, so I didn't care. I learned a lot from him, and although the situation could have been better it was what I needed to catapult to my next destination. I thought I was a late bloomer. I did not go to college right after high school; I went to work a few years before I decided to attend college. I remember talking to him about some profound things, his past, and things that had happened to me.

We wrote so much because, of course, this is 1995 through 2008, social media was in its infancy and the state and federal prison systems didn't have the technology they have today for emails and video chats. These letters were often the only means of maintaining a connection with those who were separated from us by prison walls.

I remember having to take the bus from work because I didn't have my driver's license. Unlike my siblings, who obtained their licenses at the age of sixteen, I didn't learn how to drive a stick shift, which was a requirement in our family. I became so frustrated with my driving lessons that I quit. My instructor, who happened to be my dad, said "OK" and never mentioned it again.

However, James told me that I needed to be mobile and that I needed my driver's license. He said that once I had it, I would be able to accomplish more. He was right. A few months after getting my license, at the age of twenty-one, I bought my first car, which happened to be a stick shift, for $300. I remember James telling me that he was proud of me, and that was the first time any man besides my father had ever said that to me. Now that I had a car I would visit him, and we would still write letters and talk on the phone.

On September 9, 2001, I relocated to Fairborn, Ohio, to attend Wright State University and later Antioch University, where I would spend the next eight years. James was always supportive, but let's be honest, how could he not be? He was in prison. I still had guys who I would meet for dates, but he was still there. He was my security, like an emotional blanket I carried. He would get so upset with me when I talked to him about other guys, and I was so arrogant that I didn't understand why. It was because he loved me, and I loved him as well, but he was in jail, so again, he was my emotional support. I could not believe what would happen next.

His mother passed away unexpectedly in 2003, leaving him shattered, unable to bid her farewell or find closure due to his incarceration. My heart ached for him, grappling with the agony of being separated from a loved one during their final moments. We didn't speak much during the following weeks as he was completely devastated. However, several months later, I received an unexpected check in the mail, amounting to a staggering $10,000. I was stunned and placed it on the counter, my mind racing with questions. When he finally contacted me, I became curious and asked about the source of the money, to which he assured me of its legality. He gave me a list of items to buy and do—none of which were illegal. He told me to buy a computer, so I could do my homework without having to stay out on campus or go to the library after hours. I appreciated his thoughtfulness and felt grateful that he was taking care of me. This wasn't the last time he would offer me financial support. You've heard the stories: women get with men who are in prison, the guy uses them, all he wants from them is their money. That was not my story.

We would be here all day if I went into all the intricate details, but the bottom line was I fell for this man. I was so in love with him that one of my guy friends told me he never had a chance. I asked him why we never got together, and he told me, "Your heart belonged to James, and there was no way I would set myself up for that." I couldn't believe it, but after talking to a college friend, she said the same. It wasn't love because he was in prison, but we were in love emotionally, spiritually, and romantically. People thought I was absolutely off my rocker. I would have married this man when he was released; no one could convince me otherwise. He was the love of my life.

In May 2008, I had just graduated from school with my master's degree. I was searching for a job. I was looking to relocate out of Fairborn and was ready to start my adult life. I came home from work one day to find a message on my answering machine. It was from the prison chaplain. He asked me to call him back, which I did, and he proceeded to tell me that the man that I loved so much and that I was waiting for had died. I can't tell you the devastation, the betrayal, all the things that you would think I should feel I felt. I cried and cried because I could not understand why. I waited for this man for all these years, and he died. My friend Ed told me, "James would not want you sitting around crying. You know he loved you and would not want you doing this." How many people say they have been loved by someone other than their children, parents, or grandparents? I had someone to love me unconditionally in the state that I was in then, flaws and all. Ironically, the life lessons and the hard truths he was trying to show me did not manifest until my forties.

In 2011, I was married to my now ex-husband. That year, Facebook reminded me of July 12, which would have been the birthday of my late partner, James. I shared a message on my Facebook page to express how much I missed him and how he would always be in my heart. However, one of my friends messaged me and criticized me for commemorating James, stating that it was disrespectful to my husband. I didn't think much of it at the time, since James was no longer alive. Before meeting my current husband, I knew I needed to move on from my past relationship entirely. My husband knows I had other partners before him, and he had partners before me, so it's not an issue for us. Nevertheless, I decided to get rid of the last picture I had of James and all the letters he had written to me.

Although it was a painful experience, I knew it was for the best. Sometimes, God must remove someone from our life, even if it means they pass away, to free us from the emotional attachment we have to them. James gave me the intimacy and attention I had never experienced before, but I had to let go of him to move on.

I understand that love and connection can sometimes develop in unexpected places. However, I wouldn't want my daughter to get involved in a romance with someone who is in prison. As a parent, I hope my daughter finds love in a healthy and supportive environment, free from the challenges and limitations that come with a prison romance. I will always be grateful for his lessons and wise counsel. After James passed away, and I began to get on with my life, I wish I could say I made better decisions when it came to relationships, but unfortunately, that's not how things turned out.

**LOVE IN THE FREE FUCKING WORLD!**

## FUCKING FROGS

I met a few frogs before I got to my prince or my king. One relationship was during college, and he was a 40-year-old fuck boy. I didn't realize it then because I was still in my late 20s or early 30s. Looking back, I know I did not respect him at all because he didn't take care of his children, and he would work when he needed money. It was hard to leave him alone because of the physical attraction and connection, but I saw him ten years later (that was all after I got him out of my system) and although he now had his place to live, he was still stagnant.

While we were still together, I remember my father calling and telling me that he was not suitable for me and that I needed to find someone at my level. I cried like a baby because he was telling me the truth. My father saw that he was nothing, and I thought I loved him for some reason. I met someone, we will call him Kevin: I liked his stature, attractiveness, and authoritative nature, and we became great friends. We should have remained friends because being in a relationship proved to be a disaster. He was DSM-5 certified mentally unwell, and I mean that in every sense of the word. My friends didn't care for him. My dad didn't like him at all for various reasons.

Once I began to heal, I realized that he was emotionally abusive, but at the time I was head over heels for him, and it caused the problems. He and I had many issues, so we broke up.

During this time, I began online dating and met a lovely and sweet person: Tim. He wasn't what I am usually attracted to, physically, but he was a nice guy. We got married after dating for a short time . . . very short. Surprise, surprise! My parents were beyond pissed. We had not known each other long enough to be married, but we were. Tim was a rebound, and I knew it, and I should've never gotten him involved in my mess. He was a good husband for the most part, a provider, and remembered all the occasions husbands are supposed to remember; things were good, except he did not want any children. To this day, he still does not have children.

About a year after we married, I discovered he was having an affair, which he denied. I was devastated because, up to this point, I had been wholly committed to the marriage, no matter how crazy the circumstances. We separated shortly after and I rebounded back to Kevin. I mean, who was I kidding? My heart was with him anyway. A friend called me one night. She said, "Where are you?" I was very coy, but she knew and told me that I needed to leave and go home to my husband. I did not listen. A hard head makes a soft ass. I learned the hard way.

I got pregnant, and he denied paternity, which made for a very emotionally charged pregnancy. I was shattered, and it was just a huge mess. About halfway through my pregnancy, I realized I needed to leave the home I shared with my husband. I moved back after my son was born. Tim and I attempted to rekindle the marriage, but it was broken. It was not a surprise, especially considering all that had happened, that I began divorce proceedings shortly after that. Despite everything, we remain cordial to this day. Once the divorce was finalized, we apologized to each other for all that had transpired and for the heartache we'd caused each other. Once I was emotionally healthy, I began the paternity process with Kevin. He refused to take the test, but was forced to once he was arrested and ended up serving seven years in prison for felonious assault. When he received the results, he called and asked about my son. I told him from the very beginning he was his child, but he didn't believe me. I understand why he thought he wasn't his son: I was still legally married to my husband, but I knew there was no chance he was his father. Long story short, he signed away his parental rights, which was the best thing for everybody.

I went through a spiritual process of healing the emotional scars that the entire situation had left me with. I had a male friend whom I would confide in occasionally, and he would tell me things would be OK and I would find my true love. I did not date until my son was about one. I met someone again: Brian. On the surface, he was a good guy. He treated me well until I got pregnant, and then, at that point, he ghosted me. When I told my parents I was pregnant, of course, they were upset and wanted me to be happy with the child that I had. I ended up experiencing a miscarriage. At the time, I thought it was the absolute worst thing that could ever happen to me, that my life was completely over. I did not know how to pick up the pieces and move on. I remember being in the ultrasound room, screaming at the top of my lungs because the baby was gone. My friend told me I would have a story to tell, like Job in the Bible: "Everything you lost would be given back."

Five months after my miscarriage, the revelation about Brian's deceit hit me like a ton of bricks. As I sat in front of my computer, scrolling through the damning evidence laid out by his wife on social media, I couldn't help but feel a strange mixture of disbelief and amusement. Here was a man who had duped not just me but several other unsuspecting women, all while maintaining the facade of a devoted partner.

Despite the gravity of the situation, I found myself chuckling bitterly at the absurdity of it all. How could I have been so blind to his true nature? He wasn't just a run-of-the-mill liar; he was a 50-year-old fuck boy, a man-child masquerading as a grown man.

At that moment, instead of succumbing to sadness or anger, I felt a sense of liberation wash over me. It was as if the flames of my laughter were burning away the last vestiges of my attachment to him, leaving nothing but ashes in their wake.

Driven by a newfound sense of clarity and resolve, I retrieved the ultrasound—the tangible reminder of the life that could have been—and watched as it was consumed by fire. It was a symbolic act of catharsis, a final farewell to the illusions of love and happiness that Brian had promised but never delivered.

As the flames licked at the edges of the image, I felt a weight lift from my shoulders: a sense of freedom mingled with the smoke rising into the sky. At that moment, I knew I was finally ready to move on, leaving behind the ashes of my past to embrace the promise of a brighter future. Please don't get upset with me. This is the way that I process things and let things go. I was able to let go of that trauma because I knew it was for the best. God knew the entire story and decided to shield me from it. I was very thankful.

I swore off dating after the miscarriage and decided that I needed to get myself healed, get right with God—all of the things that we try to do when our life is in a shambles. I waited about six months and decided to restart online dating. I then met a guy online named Antonio, who claimed he was a psychologist. He lived in North Carolina. My friends called him "Fake Doctor" due to some of his conversations. We talked, texted, and Skyped. We had plans to meet, but God had other plans. The weekend I was to go to North Carolina, my grandmother passed. We never met, and I ended things by texting him that he needs to be careful telling women that "God told me you're my wife."

I met a few other people after that, but nothing clicked: I wanted something else. However, I did meet a guy in the grocery store, and we hit it off. Unfortunately, our goals and expectations didn't align, so we decided not to pursue a relationship. I decided to give online dating one more chance.

I met a man who introduced himself as Jay. Initially, I was skeptical about his name since I knew it was not his given name. I questioned him (he says I interrogated him). After a month, we met in person so he could meet my father and talk with him. I wanted to do everything the right way this time. He met my parents and told them he wanted to marry me. My dad told him, "My daughter acts up. She can get crazy!"

Things moved quickly, and he invited me to his home country, where we fell in love. In September we will celebrate our seventh wedding anniversary. I remember the story my friend told me about Job, which was true. I experienced a miscarriage on September 7, 2014. However, our daughter was born on September 5, 2017, and she was my rainbow baby. She was the blessing that I never thought I would have again.

If I could offer advice to young girls and women, it would be to cherish and protect your purity for as long as possible. Waiting until marriage to engage in sexual relationships is not just about adhering to societal norms; it's about safeguarding your heart and soul.

I wish I had understood the profound impact that premarital experiences can have on our emotional and spiritual well-being. The soul ties formed through sexual encounters are real, and they can leave lasting imprints that affect how we view and approach sex in the future.

Experiencing sex before marriage can sometimes lead to a distorted perspective on sex, causing us to compare our current partners to previous ones—a comparison that is neither fair nor healthy.

It's a topic that many shy away from discussing openly, but it's essential to address. If I could turn back time, I would have chosen to save myself for my wedding night. I've realized that while societal norms may change, the timeless wisdom of the Bible remains constant.

In a world where anything goes, holding fast to the values and principles that guide us toward true fulfillment and happiness is crucial. And for me, that means honoring the sacredness of intimacy within the confines of marriage.

**THANK GOD, I AM FUCK BOY FREE!**

## SECTION IV
# FUCK JUDGEMENT

## FUCKING WEIGHT

I used to say, "I've always been big," then my father corrected me and showed pictures of me as a child, and I was nothing but legs—skinny and tall. I began to look back at other pictures and pinpoint when I started to gain weight. Fifth grade is when my weight began to spike. I don't remember much about the fifth grade, except I was the biggest and tallest kid in the class, maybe in the entire school.

When middle school rolled around, I was "thick," not fat, because my height hid my actual size. It was time for school clothes, and my mother got so frustrated because I couldn't fit the clothes from the department store, so we had to shop at the "big girl" stores, Sizes Unlimited (later called The Avenue) and Lane Bryant. What a blow! My parents bought clothes from Sizes Unlimited in the seventh and eighth grades.

My father advised me to pay more attention to my appearance, given my physical features. He wouldn't have me walking around looking like a clown, so if I had to shop at certain stores to find clothes that fit me, that's where I would shop. As a result, I kept my hair well-groomed, my attire fashionable, my face clean, and my nails neat. Although the clothes I found at those stores could have been better, I still thought some items were cute. However, one day, I walked into school and saw one of the teachers wearing the same outfit as me. I felt mortified! No middle school student wants to see their teacher wearing the same clothes. Even now, that's not a cue.

Unfortunately, there were no options for younger plus-size girls. Remember, this was 1988; the only stores that may have carried larger sizes were Lazarus, now Macy's, maybe Sears, and JCPenney—but for adults, not kids or teens. Thank God for Schottenstein's department stores, which were liquidation stores, and Marianne's.

They became my saving grace, and by the time I was a senior in high school, I was able to walk in there with the confidence that I would be able to find some cute, stylish school clothes for the year.

I am tall, 5′ 11½″, so I automatically felt like playing basketball and decided to try out for the girls' basketball team. I had to get a physical, and I weighed in at two hundred pounds, but I already knew that because earlier that week our physical education teachers took all our weights for a fitness test. Of course, I got teased, but I was used to it by then.

My doctor also took my blood pressure for the exam and told my mother it was too high (the only other time it was high was in previous chapters), so he wouldn't let me play basketball. I cried because once my father knew about my weight I would be in big trouble. Instead, he sent me to a nutritionist, which I attended a few times. I wasn't feeling it and didn't go back.

Over the years, I would sneak food and stuff myself when I ate. It didn't matter. One day, my father found out I had eaten an entire pack of hotdogs (yes, all eight); he made me run up and down the stairs in our three-story, eighty-year-old house.

We made a deal. He told me he would buy me a new dress for every fifty pounds I lost. I was on board for a few weeks and then fell off. I felt enormous! Looking back at the pictures, I was thinner than I thought. It was society and family: if you don't fit into a size 10, then you are placed into the category of being overweight.

Over thirty years ago, there were very few options, and we rarely saw plus-size people on television unless they were portrayed as clowns or jokes. However, my grandmother and aunts were plus-size women who were always well put together. When I realized that I was also plus-sized, I looked my best.

Today, we live in an inclusive society. This means those who are plus size can walk into almost any store and find something. Sidenote: Just because it is made in plus size does not necessarily mean you should put it on your body.

Plus-size women come in all shapes and sizes. I carry most of my weight around my midsection and back, so I will not wear something backless. Still, some women can confidently wear those items because they don't carry their weight in the same areas. You have to know your body shape and type.

I used to get nervous and feel uneasy whenever I was about to go out with my friends or be around many people. I didn't quite understand why I would get butterflies in my stomach or feel sick. It's ironic because I like being noticed, but only on my terms. I have always had a unique sense of style, with my love of big hair, big earrings, bright colors, and being a tall, plus-size woman. Growing up, I knew I would stand out no matter what because of my stature, so I felt I was always on display, therefore, I had to keep my "company" face on.

During my high school years, I had a difficult time as I was subjected to constant teasing because of my physical attributes, including my height, complexion, and weight. It's something that people often overlook, particularly when they have a child or teenager who is overweight. As a plus-size woman, and now a parent myself, I need to be mindful when shopping for clothes for my overweight child. Clothes that are too big or small can be uncomfortable and potentially lead to teasing from others. It is essential to ensure that pants are not too tight, shirts and pants are long enough, and that structured clothing is worn. While it is true that many of us have become more relaxed in our dress since the pandemic, wearing leggings, yoga pants, and sweats may not be the best choice for an overweight child. Trying clothes in the stores is essential to ensure they feel good and comfortable.

Additionally, it is crucial to ensure the child wears the correct undergarments, such as bras, that fit correctly. According to a 2019 *New York Times* article, 80 percent of women wear the wrong bra size, and this issue is even more prevalent among girls. Instead of wearing regular bras, many girls opt for sports bras, tank tops, and camisoles, which can be problematic.

Ensuring their hair is done is also crucial, especially for Black girls. Our culture is known for tying our self-esteem to our hair, so if an overweight child's hair is not done or cut, on top of their clothes not fitting, it can severely impact their self-esteem.

In high school, I also realized that I liked to dress up, so I made sure that I always looked nice. People would always tell me, "You are pretty to be big," or, "You are pretty for a dark-skinned girl." I didn't have boyfriends as my friends did in high school; I had boys who wanted to have sex with me, but they were never happy to be my boyfriend. I attended one dance prom, and I went with my cousin.

Once I graduated from high school, I went to work full-time, and it felt like my weight ballooned overnight; I no longer had a flat stomach, and clothes that I was able to wear months before were tight. I didn't worry about it too much because I stood on my feet at work and didn't have a car, so I caught the city bus, which meant walking about a mile round-trip every day. This approach was something I liked: it was helping me reduce my weight.

At one point, I requested from my doctor, and he gave me, something to help with weight reduction. I began, for a short time, taking a medication called Redux. It helped to some extent, and I lost a few pounds, but nothing significant. I stopped taking it because it was making me sick. I made a conscious attempt to lose weight a few years later using a Herbalife system, which involved drinking shakes and taking a handful of vitamins every day. I lost about thirty pounds in around a month, and I was excited, and walked for exercise.

Once again, this weight loss didn't last, and I regained thirty pounds, and probably twenty more. I then discovered the Atkins Diet and felt like I had hit the jackpot. I headed to the grocery store, bought all the vegetables, meat, fruit, and water I could, and began eating a carb-less diet. The weight melted away, and before I knew it, my family and friends noticed how I looked and congratulated me. Still, when I told them how, the comments were, "That is not healthy," "You are losing weight too fast," and "I hope you keep it off," which started to discourage me because I felt like I had been doing a good job. I ended up losing seventy pounds in about two months (not typical and it genuinely isn't safe).

I went to the gym at work, walked, and did exercise tapes. I was on a roll, but I got comfortable, and a few months later the weight crept back up, but I still exercised so I maintained about twenty-five pounds of it for quite a while.

In September 2001, I moved away from home and became a full-time college student. I put on the "freshman fifteen" from eating whatever at all times of the night, heading to restaurants at midnight, and doing nothing but going to school. I continued to hear from family, "You need to lose weight," "I thought you were on a diet," etc. I ignored them and continued. I counted calories and lost weight. I did SlimFast, but the best attempt I felt I made in the battle to lose weight was when I joined WeightWatchers. I had gone to the doctor because I was having pain and discomfort in my left knee. I was surprised when the nurse weighed me, and I weighed 379.8 pounds. I felt so ashamed that I had let myself get that heavy and that I was only twenty pounds away from being four hundred pounds.

I joined WeightWatchers that day, and this time I had a buddy, and we did it together. I later found out the pain in my knee was osteoarthritis—when bone surfaces become less well protected by cartilage, the bone may be exposed and damaged. As a result of decreased movement, secondary to pain, regional muscles may atrophy, and ligaments may become looser.

My doctor told me that my weight was the cause and that I needed to lose weight. I was "gung ho," I stuck to the plan, exercised, wrote down everything I ate for eight months, and lost fifty pounds. I was so excited because the weight loss was low and steady. I was weighed once a week, and it was going well until my buddy stopped attending the meetings; I still went but started to slack off with writing things down. Eventually, I stopped going altogether but maintained my weight for a while and returned to business as usual. I ended up with a bought of sciatica, which left me unable to walk, resulting in cortisone shots in my back and knee . . . NOT FUN!

Fast forward to 2010, and I found myself debating the risks and benefits of undergoing gastric bypass surgery. Despite the potential complications, I decided to go through with it. The surgery effectively reduced the size of my stomach to that of an egg. However, I realize that surgery should not be taken lightly. Afterward, I used to get sick from overeating, vitamin deficiencies, and, worst of all, dumping. Dumping syndrome is a group of symptoms that can occur after surgery to remove all or part of the stomach, or after surgery to bypass the stomach to help you lose weight. The symptoms can include nausea, vomiting, diarrhea, dizziness, sweating, and rapid heartbeat after eating, especially sweets. It occurs because food moves too quickly from the stomach to the small intestine. Managing dumping syndrome is crucial by making dietary changes, such as eating smaller, more frequent meals, avoiding high-sugar foods, and drinking liquids between meals rather than with them. In severe cases, medication or surgery may be necessary to alleviate symptoms.

One Thanksgiving weekend, I didn't feel well; I could not go to the bathroom, I became nauseated, and vomited. I spent the entire weekend in bed in agonizing pain. I ended up giving myself an enema.

Upon receiving the distressing news from the surgeon's office about my obstructed bowels, the nurse emphasized the critical nature of the situation. With a sense of urgency, she advised me to seek immediate medical attention at the emergency room should the obstruction occur again, stressing the potentially life-threatening consequences of such an event.

Shortly after surgery, I rode with my family to Atlanta to attend the funeral of my great-aunt. I asked about five times for them to pull over because I was dumping after eating some mashed potatoes at the repass. After surgery, my dad drove me back to Columbus, where I stayed for two weeks. One night, I sat and watched my parents chow down on steak, and I was in tears. I couldn't eat solid food. I was in mourning. Food mourning!

I have lost a little over 101 pounds at the time of this publication. I still have about thirty pounds to reach my goal, which is lingering, but I am confident that I will reach my goal. I take four vitamins per day. I just recently started taking the "correct" dosages for bariatric patients—if you haven't noticed by now, I sometimes have slight issues following directions (blame it on the genes!).

I still struggle with certain foods; even though the surgery has given me a jumpstart on weight loss, it is not the be-all and end-all cure. I still struggle. It gets better every day, but I want people to know that when it comes to losing weight, it is more psychological than anything else, so I am working toward my goal. I still say "fuck it" to so much now with the world we live in. As a result of the weight loss, I could conceive my children. Before having surgery, my doctor told me I would not have become pregnant at almost four hundred pounds, so I am forever grateful.

The moral to all of this is, mind your fucking business. It is not your place to badger someone about their weight. Leave them alone!

If you don't feed, fuck with, or finance them, it is none of your concern. (Thanks, NeeNe!)

No one talks about why people who have excess weight become overweight or become overly obese. It wasn't until I was in college that a nurse told me I put on all my weight so that no one would see me, therefore, I felt safe. According to the Obesity Action Coalition, the link between sexual abuse and obesity might include a desire to "de-sexualize" to protect against further abuse, as well as a range of psychiatric conditions (depression, anxiety, sleep disturbances, physical complaints, phobic reactions, low self-esteem, suicidal feelings, and substance abuse).

**FUCK THE SCALE AND SOCIETIES BEAUTY STANDARDS!**

## FUCK THE BULLIES

In the eighth grade, I began attending Columbus Bible Way Church. Even though my uncle and his family were members, we didn't know anyone else, and nobody knew us. This church differed from the one we had previously attended because I sang in the choir and attended Sunday services. My dad insisted that we go to this church. I also joined a group of middle school students who met on Sunday nights.

One day, the church's mass choir served lunch to our youth group. A choir member teased me during the event because I asked for more food. I felt upset about it and held onto this incident for years. Hearing his name would make me uncomfortable, and I would walk away or get quiet. My dad asked me why I acted that way, and I eventually told him what happened. He wished I had told him earlier, saying he would have handled the situation. I didn't enjoy my time at the church as a child due to conditions like these. Nevertheless, my parents made me go there.

I later spoke to the widow of the person who made fun of me and realized how emotional I was about it. I tend to feel things deeply, and when someone wrongs me, it affects me deeply. I had to work hard to overcome this trait. The incident was an example of how adults can tear down children. It was unacceptable for an adult to degrade and make fun of a child.

This incident was not the only one, as I had a similar experience at my previous church, Oakley Baptist. There, a girl named Kya refused to lend me her lip gloss, saying she didn't want it to be "burnt." Her comment was a dig at my complexion. Situations like these can shape how people see themselves in the world.

One of the most vivid memories I have of being bullied occurred during my fourth-grade year. I endured constant taunting and ridicule about my dark skin, height, and weight. Frustrated and determined to retaliate, I concocted a plan. I mixed Skittles with Correctol, a pink laxative from my mother's medicine cabinet, and distributed the mixture to those teasing me when I arrived at school. As a result, they fell ill, and I received a suspension as punishment. Fortunately, my father supported me, understanding the torment I had endured. Looking back, I find humor in this incident because it highlights how one can outsmart bullies without physical confrontation.

Disclaimer: Do not attempt this. Children, you will be expelled from school and face possible prosecution, and your parents could go to prison and be sued.

Sometimes, the teasing would be in my household; my brother and sister would call me "fat cow," which hurt. I lashed out by fighting and saw my weight as an advantage. If I was big I wouldn't be bothered because people would fear me. That is not the case.

The bullying finally came to a head in sixth grade. A girl, "Lena," chased me home from school. I tried to go home. My father locked me out of the house. He told me that every time she hit me, and I did not hit her back, I would get whooped with the switch. For those of you who do not know what a switch is, it is a branch from a tree or bush: this was a common item used in my household for discipline. I did not win that fight, but my father taught me a valuable lesson. You must stand up for yourself. You cannot allow people to bully you.

Standing up to bullies is a transformative experience beyond immediate confrontation. When one finds the strength to challenge an oppressor, it isn't merely a reaction to external negativity, it's a powerful affirmation of one's self-worth. Recognizing that one deserves respect and kindness, and asserting one's right to such treatment, can be a turning point in a person's perception of their value and place in the world. This act of defiance against demeaning treatment reinforces the idea that others' opinions or actions do not determine one's worth, but are inherent and immutable.

Taking a stand also fosters personal growth and resilience. Facing a bully requires tremendous courage, as the fear of retaliation or escalation can be daunting. However, individuals build a resilient spirit by confronting these fears and realizing they can overcome adversity.

Furthermore, standing up to bullies can cause a ripple effect, inspiring others to do the same and fostering a collective sense of empowerment. Witnessing someone assert their rights and demand respect can be a powerful testament to the fact that bullying should not, and cannot, be normalized. Those who might have felt isolated or defeated in their struggles can find hope and motivation in such acts of bravery. By setting this precedent, individuals uplift themselves and pave the way for others to rediscover their self-worth and reclaim their dignity. This collective empowerment creates a supportive community where individuals recognize the value in themselves and others, leading to a more compassionate and understanding society.

Since I didn't understand this as a child, the bullied became the bully for a short period. I am so ashamed that I did that, and I sincerely apologize to anyone who was on the receiving end of my bullying. I hate bullies, and that is one of the reasons that I am such an advocate for the underdog, because I was the underdog. Being an underdog is a unique and often inspiring position. When faced with significant challenges in sports, business, or personal endeavors, where the odds are stacked against you, that's when you truly learn and grow. This situation often emerges from a need for more resources, recognition, or external support, placing the underdog at a perceived disadvantage compared to more favored competitors. However, this very lack of expectation can become a source of strength. The underdog status fosters a strong sense of determination, creativity, and resilience. Without the pressure of expectations, underdogs are free to take risks and innovate, turning their supposed weaknesses into strategic advantages.

The journey of an underdog is marked by a relentless pursuit of goals, often driven by a deep internal motivation to overcome limitations and prove doubters wrong. This journey is not just about the outcome but also about the growth, learning, and character development that occurs along the way. Underdogs often become role models and sources of inspiration, showing that seemingly impossible feats can be achieved with hard work, grit, and an unwavering belief in oneself. Their stories remind us that success is not just about inherent talent or resources but also the spirit to persevere in adversity.

Educating our children, from an early age, about the importance of being kind to everyone is crucial. We never know what someone's home life is like or what obstacles they face every day. Therefore, we should not make anyone the target of our insecurities through bullying.

I have learned this lesson while teaching children with disabilities, especially those with visible disabilities. It has turned me into a protective mama bear for my students. Everyone deserves love, kindness, and respect, regardless of their differences. If you are an adult bully, it is essential to seek therapy and work on yourself. If your child is a bully, address the behavior immediately.

**FUCK BULLIES! UNDERDOGS UNITE!**

## FUCKING TRIGGERS

Triggers! "How many of us have them?" in my Whodini voice.

I had difficulty returning to Columbus after living away for fifteen years. I had built a new life in a smaller city and had no plans to return. My son and I were initially supposed to go to New York, but God had other plans for me. Returning to Columbus forced me to confront my past traumas, which I thought I had already healed from. It was tough to see the people who had hurt me, and nobody seemed to acknowledge my pain.

I started seeing a life coach to help me through this difficult time. This process taught me that I needed to forgive and let go of grudges. It was a challenging task, and I sometimes fell back into old patterns. One way of healing was writing out my issues with the person, reading it aloud as if they were in front of me, releasing my feelings into the atmosphere, and then being burned away. I also realized I needed to change my morning routine to avoid being triggered. I wasn't a morning person as a child, so being woken up was always a traumatic experience for me. My mother wasn't gentle with waking us up, which worsened things. However, if I woke up on my own, I was fine.

Similarly, my son is also not a morning person: if he is woken up, he is grumpy. But as he has grown older, he has started waking up independently. These experiences taught me a lot about myself and my relationships with others.

It turns out that having children can be one of the biggest triggers for people who have experienced trauma. An article titled "The Real Reasons You Feel Triggered by Your Child's Behavior" explains that our own traumatic experiences shape our reactions to our children's behavior. Identifying and understanding the sources of our triggers can help us start the healing process. By healing from our traumatic experiences and meeting more of our needs, we can feel triggered less often.

In my own experience, I have found that therapy and treatment can be beneficial. Unfortunately, when I was a child, therapy was not something that was acknowledged in my community or in my home. But now there are so many avenues for getting the help we need. I'm still a work in progress, and God is working it out.

> **GIVE YOURSELF SOME GRACE;**
> **LIFE IS TRIGGING AS FUCK!**

## FUCK BEING SHY

Disclaimer: I'm not a doctor or therapist. I have never been diagnosed with any type of anxiety prior to 2024.

I looked at the symptoms and came to my own conclusions. Shy, who me? Who knows?

The Anxiety and Depression Association of America discusses social anxiety disorder as follows:

> Social anxiety disorder affects approximately fifteen million American adults and is the second most diagnosed anxiety disorder following specific phobia. The average age of onset for social anxiety disorder is during the teenage years. Although individuals diagnosed with social anxiety disorder commonly report extreme shyness in childhood, it is essential to note that this disorder is not simply shyness.
>
> More than shyness: "fewer than 5 percent of people with social anxiety disorder seek treatment in the year following initial onset, and more than a third of people report symptoms for ten or more years before seeking help.
>
> Symptoms: intense physical symptoms, such as a rapid heart rate, nausea, and sweating, and may experience full-blown attacks when confronting a feared situation. Black women often find themselves in situations at workplaces, colleges, and professional school settings where they are the only, or the first ones, to achieve something. In such cases, we are taught that we must work twice as hard to get halfway ahead, that our behavior reflects on the entire racial community,

and that we face more scrutiny than our white colleagues. This is a reality that is not entirely unfounded. These beliefs, coupled with the Strong Black Woman image, increase the risk for social anxiety (Anxiety and Depression Association of America, 2009).

Another social anxiety risk factor in the workplace and college/graduate/professional school setting is the "acting white" accusation. "The "acting white" accusation (AWA) is a cultural invalidation commonly experienced by people of color that challenges their ethnic-racial authenticity for demonstrating behaviors that are not traditionally associated with their ethnic-racial group" (Durkee & Gomez, 2021).

Far too often, we forget that there are more than three (3) ways to be a Black woman in this country. The acting white accusation has nothing to do with wanting to be white and everything to do with what it means to be Black. In other words, it is an attack on one's racial identity, which, in turn, can create anxiety (Neal-Barnett, 2018).

**FUCK SOCIETY!**

# SECTION V
# FUCKING ADULTHOOD

## FUCKING COLLEGE

I decided I wanted to be a teacher. When I started I wanted to be a childcare teacher until I found out how much they make. It did not make sense, so I became a schoolteacher. I packed up everything I had, which was a little, and moved an hour away. I felt like I was out of place: I felt so old. I don't know why these are limitations I put on myself. I just knew I was twenty-four years old and a freshman in college. College was hard.

I graduated in 1995 from high school and, in 1997, I started taking some classes. It was 2001, and this was not a community college. This was not a class of twenty people. I walked into Oleman Hall, and there were 300 people in my Psychology 101 class; I did not know anybody. My sister went to school at Wilberforce University, which was about twenty minutes away. I lived in nontraditional student apartments across the hall from a young mother and her toddler daughter.

I remember one of my math classes—I worked my ass off for a C. In the same class, I can remember yelling at the traditional "Mommy and Daddy paid for college" students because they were being rude and disrespectful, while those of us who were paying for school ourselves were trying to pay attention so that we could pass the class with a good grade. I didn't go to parties. I went to some events on campus. I tried to join a sorority, but that didn't work out. All I did was go to class, go to work, come home steadily, and repeat.

In 2002, I met a woman named Michelle, and we became "Friends." She was not from the area either, and I would later learn we shared a lot of trauma, and maybe that was the basis of our friendship. But it gave me something to do outside of my routine. We had fun; her family would come, and we would go on outings, travel, etc. In hindsight, we were close, but this person wasn't indeed my friend—I will get into that later.

Being one of the few African Americans in my classes was a familiar scenario, often finding myself among just two or three others at most. The education majors especially leaned towards being predominantly white females. Despite the lack of diversity, these classrooms frequently ignited compelling discussions. We explored a range of topics, offering perspectives that were both enlightening and enriching. As a minority voice in these settings, I found value in contributing to these conversations and expanding the understanding of everyone involved.

However, there were moments of frustration. I recall one professor who, whenever issues about Black people arose, would inevitably turn to me and ask, "Ms. Gatewood, what are your thoughts?" It became tiresome, feeling as though I was expected to represent an entire race. In response, I expressed my frustration, explaining that I couldn't speak for everyone and that my experiences didn't encompass the entirety of Black experiences—I hadn't grown up in the ghetto or projects.

I struggled to find my footing with college life. I failed one class and struggled in others. It wasn't because I didn't do the work. It wasn't because I didn't have the intellect. I thought something was wrong with me. I made my way to disability services to speak with someone. I told them that I thought I had a learning disability. I met with the guy for a couple of sessions, and he told me, "Ms. Gatewood, you do not have a learning disability; you're lazy!" He said I needed to manage my time better, quit my job, and get my life together. I don't know about you, but when somebody tells you to leave your job, it is met with resistance for good reason.

I talked it over with my dad. He told me to go to bed early, get up early, go to class, make sure I tape my lectures, stay after to rewrite my notes, study outside of my apartment, go to sleep when I'm sleepy, and I needed to do things when I was fresh. I got a call center job on weekends only, which worked well. I could study and work. Before making these changes, I got myself into a health situation because I was taking No-Doze and other stimulants to keep me awake so that I could stay up all night studying. Those pills almost gave me a heart attack.

After facing some setbacks, I regrouped and began progressing towards my degree. However, in "Kia's world" fashion, I encountered another obstacle that was all too familiar to me. My academic advisor informed me that my financial aid was running out and I needed to complete my degree in the next few quarters. Feeling unsure of what to do, I investigated other majors and spoke with my advisor to find out if I had enough credits to graduate in Organizational Leadership. To my relief, I did, and so I changed my major. My previous coursework at Columbus State was counted as electives, and on November 19, 2005, I successfully graduated with a bachelor's degree.

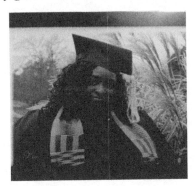

A year later I enrolled at Antioch University Midwest as an Early Childhood major because I still wanted to be a kindergarten teacher, but during orientation I noticed that there were only white women.

This meant that the oversaturation of the market meant that there would be no job for me when I graduated. I decided to change my major to Special Education, which was one of the best decisions I ever made. Our classes were enjoyable, and I met some great people. Although white women still dominated, our cohort had at least five Black women, including myself. I was thrilled and worked hard to succeed. Unfortunately, during the final quarter of my degree program, my dad fell seriously ill. But despite this challenging time, I managed to graduate in May 2008 with my Master of Education degree in Special Education.

**FUCK THAT, GET YOUR EDUCATION!**

## FUCK CANCER

Cancer has affected a few people in my family growing up. I had never seen the full effects of what this horrible disease can do to someone's body and spirit until my father was diagnosed in 2007. I remember going to my godfather's church and sitting there, crying hysterically. We had just been told that my father had multiple myeloma, a cancer that forms in a type of white blood cell called a plasma cell. Healthy plasma cells help fight infections by making proteins called antibodies. Antibodies find and attack germs. In multiple myeloma, cancerous plasma cells build up in the bone marrow. Until he was diagnosed, I had no idea what this was. I had never heard of it, and it was rare. My dad's back had been hurting for a while, but he hadn't gone to the doctor. By the time he went, that's what they told him. The first doctor told him he had months to live. Then, he decided to go to the James Cancer Hospital at Ohio State University.

My siblings and I were all away. My brother was overseas, my sister was in Georgia, and I was finishing my master's program an hour away. Nobody knows how to handle things. No manual tells you how to respond. Whose appearance has been altered by cancer. My dad ended up in the hospital. He was taking a holistic route for his treatment along with treatments from his doctor, but there were some contraindications, which caused his blood platelets to drop entirely to dangerous levels. We are supposed to have between 150,000 and 450,000 blood platelets. My father had six!

When someone's platelets drop, it causes their mental state to become altered. We thought my father was having a nervous breakdown with some of the things he was saying. It was due to the platelets. He underwent a procedure called a plasma exchange, also known as plasmapheresis, which is a way to "clean" your blood. It works sort of like kidney dialysis. During the treatment, plasma—the liquid part of your blood—gets replaced with plasma from a donor or usually a substitute like albumin.

I will never forget that smell. I stayed at the hospital for an entire weekend with my dad while they did the exchange. As his platelets returned to normal, so did his mental capacity. I was student teaching; I had about two months left and had to go, resulting in me student teaching until the last day of school before I could graduate. The great thing was that my father was well, and he was able to see me get my master's degree.

During one of his hospitalizations, I had an upper respiratory infection, so I was unable to see him when he came home from the hospital. I hadn't seen him in a while, and when I did, I was in disbelief. My sister and I were Daddy's girls; he was our hero. The strongest man in the world can handle anything, so seeing how frail he was utterly broke my heart. Every time I looked at him, I had to look away. I would go into the bathroom, or another room, and start crying. He looked like a shell of himself: at his highest height he was 6' 3½", and about 240 pounds, which was not how he looked anymore. I admit I could not handle it. I did not know what to say or what to do. It was just so hard to see him in that state.

He was able to beat it, and the cancer was gone for a few years. My son was born in 2013, and my father made it his business to build his crib. We could spend some time together before he was born, which was nice. He was so excited to have a grandson. Although the circumstances weren't the greatest, he loved him nonetheless.

Christmas 2014, Dad wasn't feeling well and was told he had some tumors. He decided to heal himself through a stem cell transplant, by harvesting his cells. Everything seemed to be working well. He was healing. His immune system was compromised, so he always wore a mask. People were told to wear masks or give him some space.

We had no idea then, but 2015 would become one of the worst years of our family's lives. On February 26, I received a phone call from my mother telling me my grandmother had passed. I was in shock, but not surprised, because she had been diagnosed with dementia and was in a nursing home—but when my mother told me that it was my grandmother, my granny Alberta, I lost it.

You see, my grandmother was the grandmother of grandmothers. She loved being a grandmother of mine; me, my sister and brother were her only grandchildren, so we got to spend time with her every weekend, and during break holidays we spent time with her. As we were growing up, she lived in the house with us, or across or down the street, so we were extremely close to her. She was fiercely protective of my father and us. I could not believe what I was hearing. My father had been calling her, and she did not answer, which was not normal, so my aunt, who lived in the same building, went with another aunt only to discover that my grandmother had died in her sleep.

I had to leave work. I picked up my son from childcare, went home, packed some clothes, and drove two-and-a-half hours to Columbus. I told my dad I would help him do everything because I knew he could not. I sat in front of her building, scared to enter her apartment, not knowing what I would find, but once I arrived it was just so peaceful and quiet. I couldn't believe she was not there. My father, being her only child, was heartbroken; their relationship was so incredibly close.

It was almost unbearable for him to be here when she wasn't. During the next few months he healed, but then something shifted. I did not know what was happening, but I felt my parents were hiding something.

The days leading up to May 29, 2015 were crazy. My cousin called and asked when I was coming to visit. I told her I would be there Friday, and she told me I needed to come sooner. I asked her why, and she told me my dad wasn't doing well. My mother was not being forthcoming. I told her I would be there as soon as I could. My brother arrived before I did, so he knew what was going on. My sister and I did not. Tuesday morning, I received a call on my classroom phone. The secretary said my mom was on the line. My stomach dropped because my cell phone was sitting there, but it was silent. She said, "Your dad said he is done! So, it would be best if you came home as soon as possible."

I didn't know what was going on. She said to arrive as soon as possible, so I had to pick my sister up at the Dayton airport before getting to Columbus, because that was the only flight she could get from Atlanta. That was the longest 85-mile drive of my entire life. I was "driving 100 on the freeway swerving" when we pulled up; my sister jumped out of the car, snatched my son up, and headed upstairs. I parked, took a deep breath, and went to his room. My cousin, whom my dad helped raise, met me in the hall, and it got real.

Nothing on this earth prepared me for seeing my father lying in that bed, almost one hundred pounds less than what he usually weighed, with black blotches all over his body. I wanted answers, and I wanted them now! I sat on the bed with my son, crying and screaming on my dad's chest, begging him to continue to fight the cancer. I was pleading with him not to give up. His doctor took a while to come in, but I could see the defeat on his face when he did.

The cancer returned with vengeance, and there was nothing more that could be done—my father, who had fought for almost nine years. I couldn't believe it was coming to an end. That day, the hospital was flooded with our family, friends, extended relatives, and church family, who came to visit. I remember our conversation while no one else was around, and he told me to live my life. I told him that I would.

He told us his plan; the plan was for him to go home to die. I spoke to the hospice nurse, who shared with me that she had never seen someone hold on as long as my father did, but he was waiting for his grandson. He wanted to see his grandchildren before he passed. My niece could not make it, but he could speak with her by phone. I couldn't sleep; my nerves were frazzled, and I prayed for a miracle.

Our former first lady at church told me, "When someone has decided that they are finished fighting, there's nothing anyone can do; no amount of praying will do once that person has said that's it, so all we can do is honor their wishes." At one point during the night, he asked for some more pain medicine. It wasn't until I saw him in that pain that I understood that he was not giving up and had fought the good fight.

The next day, he was transported home. The house was filled with people coming to pay their respects and say their last goodbyes. I called my grandfather and told him that he was dying, and if he wanted to see him, he had to come now. He didn't come by because he was ill, but his brothers arrived. I was thirty-eight years old when I saw the complete cycle of death: the death rattle, the restlessness, the smell, the stillness. My son was in the room across the hall from my dad's bed. My sister and I were headed to the funeral home. My mom called on our way back. I knew before I answered the phone when we got back that my daddy was gone. He was fifty-eight years old. He was two weeks shy of his fifty-ninth birthday and a little less than a month from his thirty-ninth wedding anniversary. It has been almost nine years, and it still is unbelievable that he is gone. Grief takes on so many different forms. You don't know how you will handle grief until something happens. His service was fantastic. My cousin took over music, and the memorial service turned into a true celebration of my father's life.

    I wrote his obituary as I did my grandmother's. I designed his program more like a small novel to celebrate who he was and let everyone else know about it. After his service, I visited my boyfriend in New York and just sat on the beach and cried. I would say that I did not start to grieve for him until months later. I know that they say there are seven stages of grief. I have probably been through each stage more than once, and I don't know if this is normal or if this is something that happens because it was a parent. I am not sure, but I don't think you will ever get over the death of a parent. I remember having a conversation with one of my aunts regarding my grandmother and her sister; she said, "Your grandmother died of a broken heart because she was unable to visit your father in the hospital after his stem cell transplant." After all, she was recovering from pneumonia. She also said, "Your dad also died of a broken heart because his mother died, and then the cancer that he fought so hard against came back for a third time." I thought about that statement many times, and she was right. Now they've both been together. It's so wild because my son was two when he passed, and he still says he misses him. I don't know what he remembers or what he doesn't. We have pictures, his YouTube videos, and the testimonials of people who met and worked with him, and it's hard to believe that he's gone. I miss both terribly. My grandmother would be in her late 80s and still be loving on her great-grandchildren. My daughter is named after her, and my niece was born the day after she passed four years later. They both impacted me and taught me what it means to be a mother and keep going even after tragedy.

**FUCK CANCER, FUCK CANCER, FUCK CANCER!**

## **FUCKING ROCK BOTTOM**

It's strange how sometimes we fail to realize the actual intensity of our emotions until we speak them out loud or put them down in writing. I remember writing the following passage a week after a painful experience in 2009. I was hoping to find some relief from the agony, to make my heartache go away. So, within twenty-four hours, I took seven Tylenol PM pills to fall asleep. I slept for twenty out of those twenty-four hours. I believed that if I stayed asleep, I would no longer feel the pain of heartbreak, disappointment, tears, or depression.

One week ago, I took those pills, and last night I prayed to God for forgiveness for wanting to end my own life and for allowing the devil to have so much power over me. I cried myself to sleep just from being sick and tired and feeling that everything was in shambles and there was no way out.

I had never felt so low in my life; even in my early years of dealing with the pain of the rape, I had never been this depressed. Even now, almost fifteen years later, I realize this was the lowest point in my life. Alone, heartbroken, empty, hopeless, and despair is what I felt, feeling that I've always gotten a "raw" deal because I was raped and endured ridicule from peers, adults, and sometimes family members because of my weight. Loveless relationships, longing to have my own family, complete with a husband and children, never to have it happen, and now I was without a job. I quit my first teaching job within three months of the start of the school year. Little to no support, depression, sadness, and loneliness had overtaken me entirely.

Even now, as I read what I wrote, I cannot believe that I was in such a desperate space that I was going to commit suicide. It's unbelievable to me, but when you are in it, you don't see any other options: whatever will make you feel better, that's what you will do.

When I tell you that my father was having none of it, he and my grandmother drove two hours to Cincinnati, Ohio, and banged down on my door. My mother called me and told me to open the door because they were not leaving. I finally did, and my grandmother came in and started cleaning up because my apartment was completely trashed. My father asked what the problem was; honestly, I don't remember what I said. I remember feeling there was no other way but God! I'm so thankful that the period I tried to write became a comma.

Please get some help; 2023 would've never happened if I would have taken my life in 2009. This is the first time I have publicly admitted this, but there is no shame now, only gratitude that the Lord saw fit to continue my story where I was trying to end it myself. Looking back, I can tell myself, "Girl . . . life was not that bad!"

If anybody is contemplating suicide and thinks that there is no other way, please talk to someone or call the suicide prevention hotline at 988.

**YOU ARE NOT FUCKING ALONE!**

## FUCKING MOTHERHOOD

If I had written this book in 2016 or even 2017, it would be filled with unflattering and unbecoming words, but because of prayer and healing, I can show grace. My mother mothered me the way my grandmother mothered her. My grandmother raised seven children, mostly independently, from the 50s through the early 80s. She raised her niece and many of my younger cousins. She was very stoic, secretive, and controlled. She never smiled, didn't like pictures of her, and, like many women of that time, she was partial to her male children and grandchildren. Her way of showing love was through food and shelter. Her house was a revolving door of her children, grandchildren, friends, and strangers. Her children called her by her first name and not "Mom." I felt like the "black sheep, problem child" due to how I was mothered—little to no affection, and no praise or encouragement from her. I vowed I would be better for my children. I pray I succeed. Once I let go of the fairytale mother I wanted and accepted the mother I was born to, I could let go of resentment and annoyance with her.

I don't know what the hell I was thinking when I decided that I was going to become a mother at thirty-six years old. I love my son, but when I tell you that I wasn't ready for everything that motherhood entails, and when I tell you that motherhood is for young women, don't give me wrong; we have children when we're supposed to, and I think that if I would've had children younger, my parents would've probably ended up raising them. Still, the fact remains, motherhood is for younger women. I had a miscarriage when my son was eighteen months old and ended up having my daughter the month before I turned forty-two. When I got pregnant with my son, I was told I was of advanced maternal age. Four years later, I was a geriatric mother.

My daughter tore my body up. She sat on my sciatic nerve for the last three months of my pregnancy. Things that happened to me with her did not happen with my son. Everything was pretty easy with him, except his delivery. His delivery was from the movies; I always wanted my father in the room when I had my children.

February 21, 2013, I was leaving Saint Elizabeth Hospital and Cincinnati. While at the stoplight, I was rear-ended by an older woman. I was on the phone talking to my sister when it happened. She told me not to move and to wait until the paramedics got there. The lady must have gotten scared because when she walked around the car and saw that I was pregnant, she panicked and immediately called 911. Paramedics arrived. I went back to the hospital I had just come from. They monitored me and the baby and said we could go home. My back was killing me, so I laid on a rice pack. I called my teammate at work and told her I would start my maternity leave one day early.

I slept so well; it was my best sleep ever, and I felt yucky. I don't remember the exact times, but I remember calling my father about seven in the evening and asking him to pray for me, and with me, because my back was hurting and I was having spasms. He did. We were on the phone for thirty minutes when my mother asked what he was doing. He told her he was praying for me. She said, "Those are not back spasms; she is in labor!" "Hang up and call 911!" were her instructions to me. I was pretty much on my own at this point.

I called 911 and told the controller I was in labor. She asked if my water had broken. I said no, and she said they would be on the way. I called my teammate and a friend who lived in Cincinnati to see if someone could get me. My water broke while I was sitting on my couch. The paramedics were there, and soon I could not walk—and here comes the dramatics. I slid across the floor on my knees to the door. I lived in a renovated mansion, so I had to open my door and the main door. I had nothing but a T-shirt. The paramedics got us into the ambulance. He pulled around the corner. One of the paramedics said, "Dude! She's crowning!" And there he was: two or three pushes and my son was born when we arrived at the hospital. He received a standing ovation from all the staff and people in the emergency room.

My teammate and her family were behind the ambulance when he was born, and she was the first one to see him. I ended up writing a thank-you note to the paramedics. I did not know their names, but I thanked them for preserving my dignity by making sure I was covered. My son came into the world with an audience and is still this way. My son shared his birthday with his great-great-aunt, and she was just tickled pink. He is highly gifted, artistic, and well-spoken.

With my daughter, I was nauseated all nine months. I could no longer wear my wedding band because my skin became utterly irritated with the metals, which had never happened before, and exhaustion became my middle name. She was such a calm baby. She was very in tune with people's energy, and when she got upset, it was for a reason—something was not right with the person. She was a happy baby and a people watcher like her namesake, Grandma Alberta. The doctors had me undergo genetic testing due to my age; she was such a lady her legs were crossed so that we could not see her gender. She was a labor of love who showed up on Labor Day.

I wasn't feeling well; I just lay around after being up all night nesting. It was 3 a.m., and my husband and son were sleeping.

I was wide awake. My mom told my husband he needed to call his boss because he was not going to be able to return to work. He tried his best to get my mother in the delivery room. I told him he made our daughter and could watch her come into the world. I had dreamed of a water birth, but at the hospital they would not allow it because of the monitor I had to wear. The nurse wouldn't let me wear my gown, that I couldn't wear with my son because it was not cut in the front, so I politely asked her for a pair of scissors and cut the gown where it needed to be cut so I could be cute, which I was. They tried to send me home before all of this, but I told them she would be born in the parking lot if I left.

I know my body, and I know my children, so every time my husband and the nurses were out of the room I would stimulate my nipples to start contractions, which worked because, after a couple of hours, I dilated enough for them to admit me. I remember my dad telling me not to let them induce me. I was scheduled for induction with her in two weeks. I sat in the room. I was able to use the balance ball while my husband watched wrestling. I was in so much pain, and I tried so hard not to get anything, but I settled on some Tylenol. Yes, I know it did nothing for the pain. Then, after it became too much, I asked for an epidural. The lady left the room and came back, door open with the needle in her hand, as if the Lord himself had said, "Not today." My daughter was coming into the world. It happened so quickly they dropped everything on the table. My husband jumped up to get ready for her delivery.

My daughter struggled to nurse. She ended up in the NICU, the neonatal intensive care unit, because she was losing weight. I had to give up my dream of exclusively nursing her for her to survive. After prayer and waiting, she came out of the NICU and we went home. My daughter's personality did not show up until she was about two years old. She is a singer, dancer, actress, and the most annoying little sister in the world, according to her brother. If you look up Margaret from *Dennis the Menace*, that explains my daughter.

Even writing it, I am exhausted. Ha! Motherhood is all-hands-on-deck if you care about how your children are raised. If you don't care, if they watch whatever they want, eat whatever they want, and go wherever they want, it's going to be so easy. But when you are breaking generational curses, generational mindsets, and cultural norms, this shit is not for the weak! My aunt, who was in her 80s then, told me that we were brave to have children in this society, and she was right. It is so scary. One of my cousins talks about missing out on spending the night for sleepovers at his friend's houses, and I told him when you have children, you will understand why your parents made that decision. I told him about the terror that you feel when your children are not with you and in somebody else's care because you can't control what's happening where they are. I said you will only understand when you have children; you will thank your parents.

I married a man from a different culture, where the women are responsible for the children and the men are responsible for providing for the family, which has caused some rips in my household because I wasn't raised that way. Although he worked a lot, my father was very involved and hands-on with us, so I automatically expected that from my husband. It's gotten better over the years, but it is difficult to "teach an old dog new tricks." Thank God for the seasoned mothers and my friends who are also mothers, because we need each other. It is so hard, but I know my children will be OK. I pray with them and ensure they're involved in church. I model what is right.

I remember my father telling me that it's not the children that have changed: it's the parents. All I must do is remember what I was taught and how I was raised. No! There is so much more going on than we ever had. Social media, computers, and phones make it so much harder to raise your children. Look out when they start reading and understanding what's happening worldwide. My son is eleven and keeps begging us for a phone. We will not allow it yet. He has a MacBook, but I have it locked down so that whatever he wants to watch or look at something, I must approve it. Honestly, I don't feel that is enough because I can control what he looks at, listens to, and reads at home, but I am not at school with or with him when he is doing extracurricular activities. My daughter is six and trying to keep her from shaking her ass and watching inappropriate videos on YouTube, and mimicking what she sees, is exhausting. There's a reason that it takes a man and a woman to have children, watch them, and raise them. Every pair of eyes you can spare is needed, which is why the village, for which I am so thankful, is needed. I don't know where I would be without my mother, friends, cousins, sister, brother, and sister-in-law.

I was so wrapped up in being a mother that I forgot who I was. I forgot what I liked and didn't like. Everything was surrounding my children, and that was something. I remember my aunt told my grandmother about my dad and that she had to have a life outside of him because he was going to grow up and leave and have a family of his own, which he did. We get so focused on making sure our children have everything *they* need that we forget everything that *we* need.

I have been a mother for eleven years, but it feels like a lifetime. I have heard people with grown children say it's harder to parent when your children are adults versus when they're children, and I can understand why. I gave my parents fits. There was a reason, and not just because I struggled with everything. If counseling had been readily available when I was a kid, I would be much better than I am now. I got advice from my friends who told me you must do this. You must set a schedule. You must make sure that they have boundaries so that they know Mommy needs space, and we do. Everyone needs their time alone. There's a reason: we must reflect, breathe, and enjoy ourselves before anyone else can. That's the hardest lesson that I had to learn. Nobody is responsible for your happiness but you. My husband asked me one time if I was happy with myself. I told him I was content, and he said he could tell. He never elaborated on why he said that, but I know why during that time. Our daughter was maybe a year old; I had gained weight dealing with the postpartum, job, and settling into our new home. So, no, I wasn't happy with myself. I am now, but it took a long time to get here.

## FUCK THEM KIDS! . . . NOT REALLY, LOL

## FUCKING FRIENDS

It's interesting to think about how our first friendships are often with our siblings or cousins and how those connections can shape who we become. As a parent, I want to raise my children to be kind and compassionate friends to others. I've had a hard time making friends because of past experiences with hurt and betrayal. I've been reflecting on this lately, and while I don't want to dwell on it too much, I mentioned one person in my college chapter who I thought was my best friend. We had plans for her to be a bridesmaid at my wedding, but things didn't work out as expected. My family didn't care for her, and my husband advised me to let it go and move on.

I received a phone call in 2020, and it was her. She was in a manic state, which is the only reason I returned her call. Once I spoke with her, I realized that she was full-blown manic and in need of some extensive mental health treatment that I could not provide. The conversations would continue for hours, with her talking 98 percent of the time. She verbally vomited for a few months, the phone calls turned into texts, and the texts went unanswered. In the year 2022, she called me again. This time, her voice sounded much brighter and she seemed to be in a better place. However, I couldn't ignore that her brilliance made it even more tragic. As time passed, I began to realize that our interactions were negatively impacting my mental health.

I felt very down; I was already dealing with a traumatic situation that had happened to me. I needed to set boundaries. I was spending most of my days talking to her on the phone. It got to be too much, in and out of mental facilities, and one day I had to rip the Band-Aid off. I told her that to get well, she would have to do right by her parents, especially her mother. I was raised to respect my parents no matter what. I have not been around anyone who talked to their mother like she did. I'm a grown woman with a husband and children, and I would never call my mother some of the names she called hers, but I digress. She didn't take this well, and I didn't expect her to. The following conversation we would have would be our last—full-blown manic again; she was engaging in some highly risky behaviors.

I recall telling her she needed help and that I would assist her when she was ready to receive it. After that, everything my father, sister, mother, and husband had told me about her came to light. She started insulting me, called me a bitch, repeatedly, and wished terrible things on my family. I was about to let it go, but I sent another message. I explained to her that I had always been a great friend and never did anything intentionally wrong to her. Despite her mistreatment of those around her, I was still willing to try and be her friend. However, at this point, my mental health and my family's well-being were more important than my friendship with her. I hope she gets help because of the things she used to do in college; her mental health diagnosis explains it all. My father always said she was jealous of me, and I could never understand why. Still, with life experience, I now realize that sometimes people envy what you have, whether material possessions or something else.

It isn't easy to trust people after experiencing a fallout in a friendship. I've become more cautious about whom I call my friend and tend to sit back and observe more. I had a friend I'd been close to since age sixteen, but our friendship hit a rough patch due to our differing religious beliefs. Though it's been a while since we've talked, I wish her the best. My friend Ed has been one of the most supportive people in my life. However, I find it challenging to maintain long-distance friendships. I work with a great group of ladies, and two of them have become close friends of mine. One is a pre-K teacher, who had my children in her class, and the other is my assistant, with whom I share a love for special-needs children. My older cousins are also close friends with whom I bond over life experiences. While I don't have many close friends, I have a handful of solid people who have shown up for me when I needed them the most. I've learned that friendships don't necessarily require constant communication, instead, the people who show up when you need them genuinely matter.

**FUCK FAKE FRIENDS!**

# FUCKING ADVICE TO MY 25-YEAR-OLD SELF

- Girl! You are exactly where you are supposed to be. You do not need ever to feel as though you are behind or late. Those you think are ahead of the game are only ahead of the game for themselves. When it is your time, it is your time.
- Age gives you wisdom and experience, and trauma provides you with insight.
- When it's your time to have children, you will have them; when it's time for you to be married, you'll be married. Rushing the process only leads to heartache, so being married for the right reasons is essential. There is nothing worse than being with someone because you are lonely.
- It's highly essential to stand up for yourself and not give a damn about what your family thinks early on. You must carve your path; what your family wants for you may have nothing to do with God's path. Many times, people project their fears onto others, or they try to deter us from doing something they wanted to do but didn't, or couldn't.
- Discovering your true friends early in life and cultivating those true friendships is crucial. It is hard to make genuine friendships as an adult.
- Putting yourself first is essential. If you don't care about yourself, no one else will.
- Trust yourself and your intuition.
- Heartbreak is temporary, but soul ties are forever. If he doesn't want you all, he shouldn't get a piece of you.
- There is always a method to the madness.
- You can't change the trauma you have experienced, but you can fix and heal yourself.

- Everyone is responsible for their healing.
- There's nothing wrong with taking your time. What is meant for you will be yours.
- Things will work out how they're supposed to because God doesn't make mistakes.
- If he wants to leave, let him go.
- How do you expect anyone else to respect you if you don't respect yourself?
- Respecting your parents will take you a long way.
- Save yourself because no one else will!
- Confidence goes further than looks.
- You are and always have been beautiful.
- Most importantly, no one can make you happy but you! Not your spouse, friends, children, etc. ONLY YOU!

## WHO THE FUCK AM I?

Self-awareness is a beautiful quality that becomes apparent when recognized. At forty-seven years old, I grappled with understanding the repercussions of sexual abuse that went well into my 30s. The decisions I made as a young adult, the friendships I formed, and the relationships I engaged in, many were all unfortunately shaped by the lingering effects of that trauma. When it comes to love, I find myself loving intensely—a trait my husband sometimes describes as overwhelming, particularly for someone deeply emotional.

I internalize many aspects of my life. When close to friends, I often find myself adopting their personalities or the collective traits of a group. For the longest time, I struggled to define myself: my voice seemed lost, and I believed I had to conform to someone else's image for acceptance. This struggle predates the influence of the Internet; back then, television and movies were my guides for how I should behave or dress. I knew my preferences, yet I'd emulate my favorite TV or movie star's actions or style.

I vividly recall an encounter with my husband when we first met. He posed a profound question: "Who are you?" In response, I recited my name, education, and place of origin. Unsatisfied, he pressed further, demanding to know the essence beyond my resume. This interrogation halted me because I didn't know who I was.

No one had ever posed such a question without readily accepting my surface-level responses; this pivotal moment occurred in 2015, sparking a continuous journey of self-discovery. Initiating a "walkabout," I confronted my true self by standing bare before a mirror for hours. In that reflection, I encountered the deepest recesses of my being—shame, hurt, hate, and torment. The rawness of this self-confrontation brought tears, as only I was confronting my truth.

Today, I can confidently answer the question without hesitation. Kia Renee Merrifield is a lover of plants, a connoisseur of tea, an enthusiast of Gouda cheese, and a fan of Mr. Rogers. I watch *The Golden Girls, The Cosby Show, A Different World,* and *Seinfeld* reruns as if they are in the new television lineup. Winnie the Pooh holds a special place in my heart as a favorite cartoon character. I revel in Ruby Woo lipstick, statement earrings, bold, colorful clothing, and unique fashion—the backdrop of smooth jazz, the 90s, and early 2000s neo-soul fuels my creativity. Hip-hop of OutKast and No Limit get me going at the gym while Teena Marie and Earth, Wind, and Fire provide the soundtrack in my kitchen. I relish driving down the highway with music blaring, singing show tunes from *Dream Girls* and *Rent* at the top of my lungs. I find joy in crafting unique items and home decor. Glitter, whether purple, sequined, or fur, captivates me.

I am a woman who cherishes intimate spaces over crowds. I find solace in steaming hot bubble baths scented with fresh eucalyptus and roses. Sitting on my porch at dawn, watching the sunrise while hearing distant wind chimes, is a cherished ritual. As an older mother, I love crafting and baking with my children, nieces, and nephews. A caregiver at heart, I express my love through food and care. As a fiercely passionate educator, I unwaveringly advocate for underserved students and voiceless adults.

My love for family extends to creating cherished memories, whether on the beaches of Antigua or during road trips with my children. The sound of children singing, especially my daughter, moves me to tears. I savor the aroma of newborn babies and the warmth of a heated blanket on chilly nights. With a big heart and a warm smile, I am not hesitant to use my tongue as a sharp weapon when wronged. The intricacies of my identity and experiences could go on endlessly.

**THIS IS WHO THE FUCK I AM!**

## GOING FUCKING FORWARD

I'm a woman who experienced the scare of a lifetime, and through that experience, I discovered "me," recognizing what had been holding me back and why. Saying "fuck it" is a candid expression of surrender, a momentary release from the shackles of overthinking and societal expectation. It signifies a decision to relinquish the weight of perfection, embrace life's unpredictable nature, or confront a challenge with audacity. While occasionally perceived as reckless or impulsive, this mantra can often act as a liberating affirmation, enabling individuals to break free from paralyzing indecision or fear of judgment. In these two words, there's an acceptance of life's imperfections, a willingness to embrace the unknown, and a nudge to prioritize one's own well-being and desires over external pressures. By adopting a "fuck it" attitude, individuals permit themselves to prioritize their happiness, well-being, and desires above external expectations.

However, it's essential to recognize that while this approach can be empowering in many situations, there may be times when a more measured or considerate approach is necessary. It's all about finding the right balance and ensuring one's decisions align with long-term goals and values.

Disclaimer: I'm not a doctor or therapist. I have never been diagnosed with social anxiety. I looked at the symptoms and came to my conclusions. Between these pages are my experiences with the medical world and life. I pray that you will listen to your body, assert yourself in your care, and have the courage to keep pushing through the pain and trials of this life. Don't be embarrassed by mental, physical, and emotional health struggles that have plagued our community and families for years. We're overcomers!

**FUCK EVERYTHING THAT SEEKS TO DESTROY!**

# ABOUT THE AUTHOR

Kia R. Merrifield comes from the bustling city of Columbus, Ohio, where she grew up in the tight-knit Hilltop neighborhood. As the oldest child of T. Wayne and Dorothy Gatewood, Kia learned the values of resilience, determination, and compassion from a young age. Kia is a proud graduate of West High School, where she started her journey of academic excellence. Her quest for knowledge led her to pursue a degree in Organizational Leadership from Wright State University, where she honed her leadership skills and passion for creating positive change.

Driven by her commitment to educational equality and inclusion, Kia earned a Master of Special Education from Antioch University Midwest. With knowledge and a heart for service, she embarked on a fulfilling career as an educator, touching the lives of countless students and inspiring them to reach their full potential.

Apart from her roles as a wife, mother, daughter, sister, and friend, Kia proudly wears many hats. As an aunt, niece, creator, and author, she embraces creativity and innovation in all aspects of life. But above all, Kia identifies as a survivor—a testament to her strength, resilience, and unwavering spirit in the face of adversity.

Through her writing and advocacy work, Kia seeks to uplift and empower others. She shares her journey of triumph over adversity and spreads a message of hope, resilience, and self-discovery.

*Still having the "FUCK ITS"?*

*Coming soon . . .*
*A CASE OF THE F&$!#%k ITS! (Teachers' Edition)*

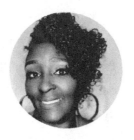

## FOLLOW ME

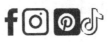

**@CASEOFTHEFITS**

STAY IN TOUCH WITH ME.
FOLLOW FOR THE LATEST
UPDATES, TIPS, GIVEAWAYS, AND
MUCH MORE!

# REFERENCES

Anxiety and Depression Association of America. (2009, October 19) *Social Anxiety Disorder*. ADAA. Available at: https://adaa.org/understanding-anxiety/social-anxiety-disorder (Accessed April 2, 2024).

CBS News. (2020, December 1) *Teacher From Roselle Won't Even Let A House Fire Stop Him From Teaching His Students Remotely*. Available at: https://www.cbsnews.com/chicago/news/teacher-from-roselle-wont-even-let-a-house-fire-stop-him-from-teaching-his-students-remotely/ (Accessed April 20, 2022).

Colizza, C. (2019, July 10). Are 8 Out of 10 Women Really Wearing the Wrong Bra Size? (Published 2019). The New York Times. https://www.nytimes.com/2019/07/10/style/lingerie-are-8-out-of-10-women-really-wearing-the-wrong-bra-size-a-bra-myth-busted.html

(2022, September 20) *Plasmapheresis and Plasma Exchange*. Available at: https://my.clevelandclinic.org/health/treatments/24197-plasmapheresis-plasma-exchange (Accessed April 2, 2024).

Durkee, M. I., & Gomez, J. M. (2021, December 9) "Mental Health Implications of the Acting White Accusation: The Role of Cultural Betrayal and Ethnic-Racial Identity Among Black and Latina/o Emerging Adults." in *American Journal of Orthopsychiatry*. 2022; 92(1): pp. 68–78. Available at: https://www.ncbi.nlm.nih.gov/pmc/articles/PMC8831462/ (Accessed June 2, 2023).

Lumanlan, J. "The Real Reasons You Feel Triggered by Your Child's Behavior." in *Psychology Today*. Available at: https://www.psychologytoday.com/us/blog/parenting-beyond-power/202402/the-real-reasons-you-feel-triggered-by-your-childs-behavior (Accessed March 2, 2024).

(2023, September 2) *Multiple myeloma: Symptoms and causes.* Available at: https://www.mayoclinic.org/diseases-conditions/multiple-myeloma/symptoms-causes/syc-20353378 (Accessed April 2, 2024).

National Institute of Mental Health (NIMH). (2022) *Social Anxiety Disorder: More Than Just Shyness.* Available at: https://www.nimh.nih.gov/health/publications/social-anxiety-disorder-more-than-just-shyness/index.shtml (Accessed October 22, 2023)

Neal-Barnett, A. (2018, April 23) Anxiety and Depression Association of America, (ADAA). Available at: https://adaa.org/learn-from-us/from-the-experts/blog-posts/consumer/be-female-anxious-and-black (Accessed August 10, 2023).

Stevelos, J., & White, C. (n.d.). *Sexual Abuse and Obesity - What's the link?* Obesity Action Coalition. Available at: https://www.obesityaction.org/resources/sexual-abuse-and-obesity-whats-the-link/ (Accessed December 2, 2023).

WellandGood.com. (2017, November 9) YouTube: Home. from https://www.wellandgood.com/social-anxiety-symptoms-black-women/amp/ (Accessed August 10, 2023).

Made in the USA
Middletown, DE
14 July 2024